THINK Yourself® CLEAN

From The Inside Out

The D.N.A. System to Reprogram Your Brain for Optimal Wellness

by

Nathalie Plamondon-Thomas,
Amazon No.1 Best Selling Author,
Founder of the THINK Yourself® ACADEMY

Tosca Reno,
New York Time Best Selling Author,
Founder of the Eat Clean® revolution,
Gemini Award Winner

THINK Yourself® CLEAN from the Inside Out

Disclaimer: The information in this book is for entertainment purposes only and does not constitute health advice in any way. Readers should consult with their own medical professionals before embarking on any health or mindset training.

Published by THINK Yourself® PUBLISHING.
www.thinkyourself.com

The author of this book can be reached as follows:
Nathalie Plamondon-Thomas:
www.dnalifecoaching.com

Tosca Reno:
www.toscareno.com

ISBN: 978-1-7753653-6-5

First Edition: July 2018

FOREWORD

August 1992. Nathalie had just moved out of her parents' house to live in her own apartment and attend high-school in a different city. That was when she discovered Costco. She had no idea you could buy full boxes of chocolate bars. This was a revelation she took full advantage of eating one or two every day during her college years.

Ten years later: She was part-owner in a printing business with over fifty employees. On her way to work Nathalie would buy three or four dozen doughnuts for her staff. She would eat some herself on her way to work, for breakfast.

December 2015. She is standing in her kitchen at 7:00 a.m., eating the remaining three portions of dessert from the night before. Suddenly, she hears a noise. Somebody is up. She quickly puts what is left back and wash the spoon to make the 'evidence' disappear.

Tosca got herself into trouble when, as a lonely young mother in a faltering marriage, she would end every day digging into a gallon of ice cream. She would spend entire days along with her children, often in new cities while her executive husband built his career. She felt isolated and miserable. Her ice cream filled evenings were the "treat" she looks forward to at the end of the day. She ate mindlessly, never comprehending that the more ice cream she ate, the more miserable she became until one day the scale flashed 204 pounds before her eyes and she realized she was obese. Every brief moment of ice cream indulgence only delivered temporary happiness. What came after were misery, ill health and depression. This was Tosca's wake up call.

These are our true stories of overeating and unhappiness. We know exactly how you feel and just like you, we enjoy our treats. However, we want more wellness for ourselves, just as you do. We are all in this together.

Through our personal journeys, we have developed practical strategies to help us stick to our wellness goals. We will teach you these strategies so that you too will have the ability to resist when the temptations seem too great!

Enjoy.

Nathalie & Tosca

TABLE OF CONTENT

PART 1

THE INTRODUCTION

CHAPTER 1:

WHAT WILL YOU GET OUT OF THIS BOOK?

*"Better keep yourself clean and bright;
you are the window through which you must
see the world."*

– George Bernard Shaw

CAN YOU REALLY THINK YOURSELF® CLEAN?

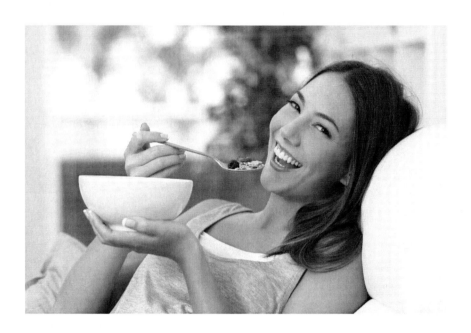

3

How hard do you have to think to become CLEAN from the inside out? How is that possible? What does the term mean? You may feel that being clean and healthy is only for others. Maybe you have an unconscious belief that, no matter how motivated you might be, you are just not able to commit to living a healthy lifestyle. This book will to teach you how to change these limiting beliefs, teach you about being CLEAN itself, and how to program your brain to reach the heights to which you have always aspired.

It is no secret that the mind and the body are connected. The brain, being one of the most complex structures in the universe, has been the subject of studies and research for years. This book will teach you the neuro-science behind reprogramming your thoughts, which will become.

THIS BOOK IS FOR YOU IF YOU:

- feel you are not clean and healthy

- feel you can't do it because it's too complicated

- don't know how to cook so you won't be able to prepare clean food

- think it's too expensive

- think that healthy food tastes terrible

- worry that you won't be able to eat what you want

- travel and eat out a lot so you feel can't control what you eat

- think it's difficult to get some of the ingredients

- feel you will have to deny yourself the foods you really want

- eat your emotions

- are addicted to certain foods (sugar, alcohol, refined foods)

- believe you don't have the right genetics

- are seeking a path to wellness

- feel that you are doing everything "right" and yet, aren't seeing results

In this book, you will learn about the D.N.A. System that Nathalie uses with her clients, combined with the expertise and wisdom of Tosca Reno, Founder of the Eat Clean® Diet, BSc., BEd., NTP, PTS, New York Times Best Selling Author. Nathalie has combined her experiences as Business Owner, Sales Manager, Fitness Professional, Speaker, Nutrition Specialist, Life Coach, Pro Trainer and Master in Neuro Linguistic Programming, into a system that will show you how to reprogram your brain to be clean and how to stay on the right track for good.

Tosca Reno has helped millions achieve optimum wellness by solving weight problems, not by diet, but instead by solving nutrition problems through Eating Clean®, a lifestyle method of managing weight and wellness.

Collectively, we will share many examples with you how our clients have become successful in changing their lives from the inside out. It is a book about 'working in' vs. 'working out'.

In this book, we will review the components of being clean and living a healthy lifestyle and help you define exactly what this means for you, in a way that will help you see the concepts differently, in a more mindful way. You will discover why your previous attempts to be healthy may not have been as successful as you would have liked. In your DNA are the fundamental and distinctive characteristics qualifying who you are. Our most profound belief is that everybody has everything they need inside themselves to succeed. It is in your DNA. Somewhere inside, you know exactly what to do in order to be your best.

We believe everybody is extraordinary and unique. Everyone can achieve the life they desire. The know-how is all within you, waiting to be discovered. Our genetics are not our fate as previously thought. Through lifestyle, nutrition and thoughts, you can affect the expression of your genes in a different way.

There are various reasons why people want to be clean and healthy and there are many elements of a healthy lifestyle. In reading this book, keep in mind you can apply our system to your health, whatever health means to you. People associate the word clean with different priorities.

Tosca worked with a woman who was so numb in her own life, she had to have a whole tray of brownies under her before she went to bed. She was eating them during the night and would wake up with an empty tray, completely unaware that she herself had eaten every last brownie. She was numb, eating her emotions. She would wake up in the morning and think: "Where did the brownies go?" She was completely unaware that she was doing this. Working with Tosca helped her realize that she unconsciously was trying to make herself ugly and create a barrier for people to not be able to hurt her. Now she has taken herself out of numbness and into caring and living. She is now present in the experience of eating and savours every bite of healthy food. Where she had used food to numb herself in the past, she has now corrected that negative behaviour and is healing herself with healthy food instead.

The vast majority of people are unhappy with their health. Since most of the population is in a health crisis, it is difficult to make a list of who these people are. We should let the statistics speak for themselves. Statistics show that one in five young people are obese in North America and that nearly two thirds of the population is overweight and/or obese. For context, this number is ten times higher than those classified as obese forty years ago. Sobering statistics show the following: (ref. The World Health Organization)

- In 2016, more than 1.9 billion adults aged 18 years and older were overweight. Of these over 650 million adults were obese.

- In 2016, 39% of adults aged 18 years and over (39% of men and 40% of women) were overweight.

- Overall, about 13% of the world's adult population (11% of men and 15% of women) were obese in 2016.

- The worldwide prevalence of obesity nearly tripled between 1975 and 2016.

The condition of overweight is accelerating world-wide. This is partly because you live in an obesogenic society - meaning you live in a world that makes it easy to access unhealthy, weight gaining foods, while physical activity has been removed from most schools. This means that only one third of you are at a lean, healthy body weight.

It is not difficult to find evidence of this. One does not need a science journal to point it out. Observe what you see in your daily life as you go about your business. The school bus driver is overweight. When you visit the hospital, a place where wellness ought to prevail, many of the health care providers are among the most overweight. No one is exempt from this plague. At the moment, 70% of the North American population is overweight or obese. Overweight and obesity are defined as "abnormal or excessive fat accumulation that may impair health." Overweight is a BMI (body mass index) greater than or equal to 25 while obesity is a BMI greater than or equal to 30.

The condition of carrying excess weight brings with it illness, including heart disease, stroke, high blood pressure, diabetes, certain cancers, gall bladder disease, gallstones, gout, respiratory problems, including sleep apnea, arthritis, inflammation, to say nothing of depression or worse. Simply put, obesity means you have an increased risk of developing disease. The cancer rate will be one in two by 2020.

Consider also that many young people are looking for ways to numb their MIND. Some people use substances, including drugs and alcohol, to numb themselves. In this century food also, has become one of these numbing substances. Many people, unable and unwilling to handle their emotions, consume food, particularly sugars and refined carbohydrates, as a way to tune out. More and more, with ready accessibility to cheap carbohydrates and refined sugars, people fill their voids in life this way. Consuming excess sugar readily becomes an addiction – alcoholism is just another form of sugar addiction. It is not a stretch to suggest that sugary foods are addictive in the same way that alcohol is addictive.

KEY CONCEPTS:

This book is for you if you are seeking the path to wellness, if you feel that you are not clean and healthy, if you feel that can't do it because it's too complicated, that you don't know how to cook so you won't be able to prepare clean food, you think it's too expensive, you think that healthy food tastes terrible, you worry that you won't be able to eat what you want, you travel too much and eat out a lot so you feel can't control what you eat, you think it's hard to get some of the ingredients, you feel you will have to deny yourself the foods you really want, you eat your emotions, you are addicted to certain foods (sugar, alcohol, refined foods), you believe you don't have the right genetics to be lean, are seeking a path to wellness and you feel that you are doing everything "right" and yet, aren't seeing results.

CHAPTER 2:
THE BOOK LAYOUT

*"The founding fathers were not only brilliant;
they were system builders and systematic
thinkers. They came up with comprehensive
plans and visions."*

Ron Chernow

The book is divided into seven major sections. The introduction, definitions of clean and healthy, the factors causing us to fail, the foundation of the system as a general overview and one section for each step of the D.N.A. System to go deeper in details.

This system is a key element of the THINK Yourself® Series. The first thing to do is to assess what you want in your kitchen or eating environment. Make a folder with floor, countertop, cupboards, backsplash, tile, paint chips samples, etc. That's the DESIRE part of the D.N.A. System: deciding exactly what you want: your vision of the new room.

Your folder is a great step and, although absolutely necessary in order to get started on the new kitchen, it is still just a folder. You cannot cook nor entertain people in a folder. In reference to selling, you probably have or know people that have already done "The List" or wrote "SMART goals" or made a "Vision Board" which are powerful tools to help you start the process. They are just incomplete. Once you have your folder, your plan, your vision board, your list, you want to implement it and transform it into a real 'kitchen' where you can cook and entertain friends.

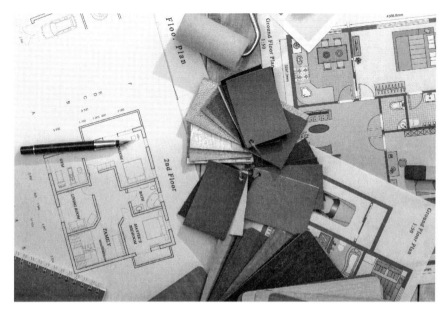

The problem that most people run into at this stage is that they try to install the new cupboards over top of the existing cupboards or stack the new countertop over the old one. You can see this doesn't make sense. The second step, before installing the new cupboards, will be to get rid of the old ones that are not serving you anymore. Demolition and gutting out the old kitchen needs to be done before putting the new cupboards in place. That is the NEW YOU part of the D.N.A. System. You clean up and get rid of old, unwanted emotions, behaviours and limiting beliefs in order to make room for what you want to implement in your life.

Once clear and empty, all you need is to fill your kitchen with brand new cupboards and furniture, new paint, new floors, and whatever you have decided in your plan. The implementation of the desires into your New You, is the ACTUALIZE part of the D.N.A. System.

The first step is to learn how the brain works and discover what you want. Then you need to clean up, and finally you can install the new desires. You will discover the complexity and power of the brain and how to elicit what you want (desire). You will learn how to make room for what you want and you'll also learn techniques to clear any negative impact from your past (new you). Finally you will learn how to program your brain with what you want (actualize).

The D.N.A. System stands for: DESIRE - NEW YOU - ACTUALIZE.

You will get a chance to practice the concepts right away in this book. We have included some brain exercises and techniques to start reprogramming your brain immediately. Tosca and Nathalie have adapted some techniques that they have employed successfully with their clients, into simple processes that you will be able to use on your own. The exercises are there to help you start "THINKING Yourself® CLEAN" right away.

You'll be amazed by your results as you apply what you discover in this book. Take the time to complete the exercises with care and thought. After all, we suspect that this may not be the first book or tool you've purchased to reestablish your health. By making a commitment to embracing these exercises and this new way of thinking, this book will be the pivotal one in your life!

If you prefer to write your answers separately, you can download our free *THINK Yourself® CLEAN from the inside out* workbook at www.thinkyourself.com.

KEY CONCEPTS:

D.N.A. SYSTEM

Desire. New You. Actualize.

Decide what you want. Make some room. Implement your dreams.

Being healthy is an inside job.

CHAPTER 3:

PERFECTLY IMPERFECT

*"Once you accept that we're all imperfect,
it's the most liberating thing in the world.
Then you can go around making mistakes and
saying the wrong thing and tripping over on
the street and all that and not feel worried."*

- Paloma Faith

It is foundational to our success in every area of life to allow ourselves to be perfectly imperfect. This book is designed to elevate you and make you feel awesome so you can reach your healthy lifestyle goals. Remember that whatever you discover in the next chapters will take you to the next level. Forget about the past. Whatever your journey, it was perfect. Whatever bad habits you used to have, they are now in the past. Make a fresh start and evolve with the premise that whatever you do next will also be perfectly imperfect.

We are not promoting a perfect, one hundred percent state of "clean" all the time. We just teach you how to aim for it, so you can be 'good' most of the time. A healthy lifestyle can co-habit with talent and life purpose. For so many women, just *being* is all they know. That was a strategy that worked up to now. It was a way of living but not necessarily the best way. You are often so cluttered with the ideas of what your life should be that it is not clear in your mind, what your true potential is. Take yourself from obvious to sublime! You were born with a divine architecture. You have the opportunity to uncover a deeper sense of self and explore what you are as a whole.

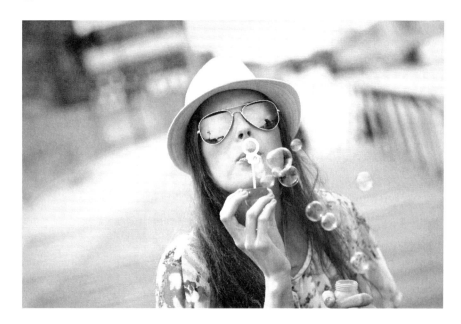

New York Times bestselling author Michael A. Singer puts it plainly in his book *The Untethered Soul,* in which he refers to the negative things you constantly say to yourself. He challenges you to consider what it would be like to free yourself from your self-imposed limitations. In this book, we will help you realize the answer to that question.

> *What you believe will be so. - Bruce Lipton,*
> *The Biology of Belief.*

See your beauty and strengths. A strong Sense of Self and a positive Self-Identity will support and fuel your present and future success in all areas of your life. By the end of this book, if you give yourself permission to commit to this process fully, you will experience positive change. You will experience a greater sense of freedom and more power over your choices. You will have a stronger and clearer vision of your New You, and you will have the tools to take you there!

Most problems are lifestyle related, which means you can address them by changing your mindset so that the behaviours will follow. The good news is you can reverse the impacts of your negative past behaviours by merely changing your thoughts. You aren't a victim of your behaviours. Your identity is very different from what you do. You are not your behaviours. By working on your mind and your identity, your behaviours will follow. In changing your thinking, you can become whatever you want to be. Your governing thoughts are not your fate.

Becoming clean and healthy is an inside job. What you believe to be true about yourself is projected onto the world around you, and then reflected back. This inner work is VITAL to your outer experience. You do not have to give your power away to outside influences. You can grab hold of the reigns and design a life that is uniquely yours. Life will provide challenges and sorrows however, you can learn the skills to transform those challenges into gifts. You can train yourself to stop, pause and reset, pick up the pieces, and move forward. Often your greatest obstacles are your best teachers, as you come to learn just how resourceful you can be, how much grit you possess, how brilliant you can be once you get out of your own way.

You are reading this book as a seed of hope through which to change your life.

The goal of the first chapters was to give you hope. You are now entering the rest of the book, which will teach you the neuro-science behind brain reprogramming and life transformation.

KEY CONCEPTS:

PERFECTLY IMPERFECT

Leave the past in the past. See yourself for who you are and trust that this journey of discovery will lead you to who you want to be.

CHAPTER 4:

FOCUS & BALANCE

*"I believe that being successful means
having a balance of success stories across
the many areas of your life. You can't truly be
considered successful in your business life if
your home life is in shambles."*

Zig Ziglar

Dedicate your focus. This book will take you on a journey to success, inviting you to reflect on yourself in a deep way, offering you processes, activities, tips and tools to use as you climb. This chapter will allow you to split your life into eight segments. You will be able to identify yourself as a Clean person in many areas of your life. We recommend for you to work on one component at a time.

*"You can do two things at once, but you can't
focus effectively on two things at once."*
– Gary Keller

Imagine a professional baseball game where a ball was just hit into the far-left field. The player focuses on the ball, runs to it and catches it in time to strike out the batter. Now change one component of the game. Pretend that twenty players will be batting at the same time towards the left fielder. With twenty balls coming at him, even the most gifted player will only be able to catch one or two balls. Can you see the chaos?

19

If people have too many balls to catch, they will inevitably drop them. People who want to make changes in their lives start off highly motivated but often with too many goals at once— change career, start a business, lose weight, get divorced, quit smoking and so on. If you try to address everything at once, failure is the result. You become overwhelmed, which leads to feelings of disappointment and potentially, depression. Your brain reminds you of these negative feelings when it hears the words clean living, eating well or exercising.

> *"Multi-tasking is great in the kitchen when you are trying to time the chicken to be ready at the same time as the potatoes. But do not assume it is a great way to manage a workday."*
>
> — *Joanne Tombrakos*

The following exercise will help you with dedicating your energy to one goal. By doing one thing at a time, you will have a much greater chance of getting positive results than if you try to change everything at once.

If you prefer to write your answers separately, remember that you can download our free *THINK Yourself® CLEAN from the inside out* workbook at www.thinkyourself.com.

DIVIDE

You are now invited to divide your life into eight segments. While you may think that your life is separated into two—work and family—there are numerous areas that influence your life. There seems to be a misconception about the word BALANCE. Since most people think there are two components, family and job, isn't it uncanny that everybody talks about finding balance between these two things and nothing else?

Think of your life as a pie chart with many slices; such as career, love life, family, health and so on. It might be that one area of your life (one slice) doesn't make you happy and this will interfere with your healthy lifestyle. Rate each area of your life from 1 to 10, reflecting how happy or not you feel in those sectors. A rating of 1 means little or no happiness. A rating of 10 means maximum happiness. If you unveil an area that's only 3 or 4 out of 10, you might choose to fix this area before you start your success plan. Work on one area at a time. If a wheel isn't balanced, the ride will be bumpy. Remember to write the numbers that you feel best represent your current state. Avoid thinking about what others would think your number should be.

For instance, a woman who does not have a significant other gave herself a 10 for *Love and Romance*. She was absolutely fine being by herself. That was okay for her, in her representational system, at that time of her life. If we had asked her mother, the mother would have probably given her a 1 out of 10 for *Love and romance*. It is not about how other people feel about each segment. It is about YOU. The same idea applies to a client who was making $25,000 per year who gave herself 8 out of 10 for *Money*. That was all she needed in her own model of reality as a humanitarian travelling the world.

Feel free to rename the segments if the label provided doesn't fit for your life and you would rather see something else there. The top part of the wheel, including Fun & Recreation, Love & Romance, Personal Growth, Health & Fitness, are connected to the primary needs of a human being, while the bottom represents other areas of human life. These are important but not as vital.

Addressing the top part of the wheel is often a priority when working with this tool. Usually, when you fix your primary needs, the other areas of life can be met naturally as a by-product. For example, if you try to work on your environment or your career (which are two segments from the bottom part of the wheel), it may be difficult to focus on these if you are violently ill (Health and Fitness) or married to someone who is not being respectful (Love and Romance). Working on Love and Romance, Health and Fitness, Personal Growth, and Fun and Recreation will very often result, as a by-product, in embellishing the rest of the wheel. All the money in the world with the nicest house and the best career in the world will not make you happy if your primary needs are not met.

Once you have given a number to each segment, make a line representing the number, and colour the area from the centre of the wheel up to the line. That will look like this:

Pretend that you are a truck and that you roll on these wheels. Do you think that the road might be a little bumpy? The bumps in your journey are caused by imbalances in the different areas of your life. It is because of these differences that deceptions and dissatisfaction are troubling.

THINK Yourself® BALANCE WHEEL

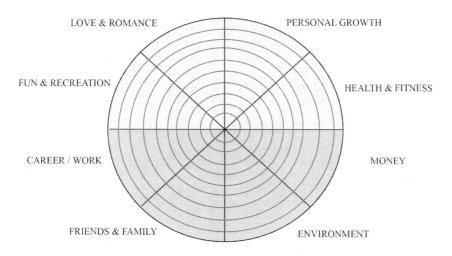

Now think about your results and have a closer look at each segment. Try to identify the connections between each one. Because this book is about clean leaving, let's focus on the health and fitness segment of the wheel. Which segment is connected to it? Let's say that if you work on your personal growth, you'll acquire the skills you need to achieve your career goals, and then your money segment will also be affected. Or if you get out of an abusive relationship, you might find the self-confidence you need to make better choices. Or if you take more time for friends or health and fitness, you will reduce stress. You may have a much more pressing matter to address before being able to focus on your clean living.

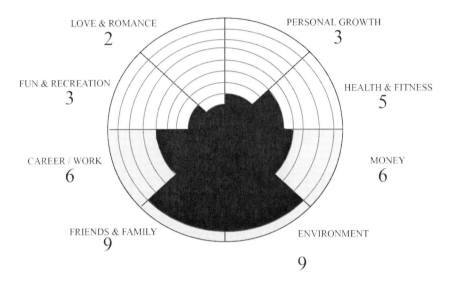

Think Yourself® BALANCE WHEEL

LOVE & ROMANCE
2

PERSONAL GROWTH
3

FUN & RECREATION
3

HEALTH & FITNESS
5

CAREER / WORK
6

MONEY
6

FRIENDS & FAMILY
9

ENVIRONMENT
9

Some areas influence others. Which area(s) of your wheel influence(s) your health?

_____

Which one do you want to address first?

_____

Now that you have identified which area of the balance wheel you want to work on, you are now ready to determine what you want and what your desired outcome is regarding this area of your life.

Visit our website www.thinkyourself.com to download our free assessment wheels.

Now that you have identified what segment of your life influences your health, let's look at being clean. What does this mean?

KEY CONCEPTS:

DEDICATE

Focus on one thing at a time. Address the main area of your life first, choosing the one that will have the most impact on the other segments. When answering the questions and doing the activities presented in this book, remember to stick to that one area of your life. Once completed, you can then address something else and re-do the exercises, answering other areas of your life.

PART 2

CLEAN
FROM THE INSIDE OUT

CHAPTER 5:

WHAT IS GOING ON?

"We struggle with eating healthily, obesity,
and access to proper nutrition for everyone.
But we have an excellent opportunity to get
on the right side of this battle by beginning to
think differently about the way that we eat and
the way that we approach food."

- Marcus Samuelsson

Managing weight through dieting is a relatively new practice for mankind. In the hunter-gatherer days, it was good day when food was available. Storing it for times of famine and eating it when available were strategies for survival, no dieting required. Food was a necessity and a pursuit required if man was to be successful. A calorie found in traditional times, was a calorie hard won and never squandered.

The past decades have born witness to dramatic shifts in the food landscape. Calories are plentiful in most places on earth. Yet, never has there been such illness. While calories are plentiful the population is at the same time, strikingly undernourished, as a result of the numerous and varied diet trends that have transformed food into an agent of demise. Hardly a week goes by without reference to the newest eating trend, super food, calorie/point weight management system. Food has become the enemy. You are gluten sensitive or intolerant. You are lactose intolerant. Peanut and other foods are now lethal pathogens. Food is suspect.

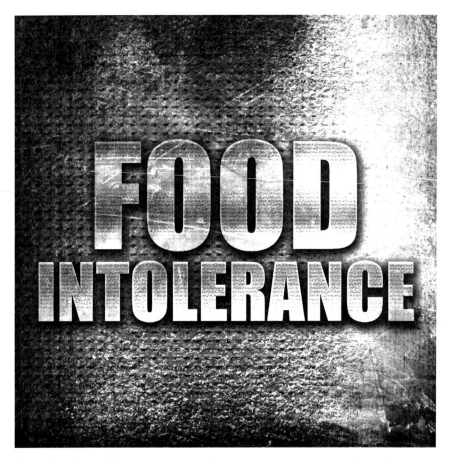

Couple this with the strange behaviors you have adopted in the pursuit of a lean physique. Diet trends have ranged from the ridiculous to the bizarre. Think back to the Cabbage Soup Diet, in which only cabbage soup is eaten for weeks on end. And for the bizarre, consider that toilet paper is often mixed with peanut butter to stay slim. The goal of losing weight at all costs may lead to paying the price with ruined health.

In an unbelievable irony, while there are so many calories to be had that overweight and obesity are commonplace in much of the world the population is overwhelmingly ill and undernourished, yet there are still many parts of the glove where being underweight is a daily truth. In India, 50% of girls and 58% of boys are underweight.

Globally, 192 million are moderately or severely underweight, to say nothing of the eating disordered.

Think also of the fact that our environment is dramatically different than what it once was. Today, studies reveal that more deaths occur from environmental factors than ever before.[1] As the study reveals, "as many as 9 million deaths were caused by diseases from toxic emissions." And polluted air is not the only culprit. Contaminated water is also to blame. This death toll means that 1 in 6 premature deaths was from pollution. That is more than smoking, hunger, natural disasters, AIDS, tuberculosis and malaria combined!!

Not only does the environment alter our human wellness within the planetary space, it alters the very foods harvested from it. If acid rain falls on a crop it ultimately fouls the plants that form food. If air quality is diminished, the resulting plants and food grown in that environment is similarly diminished. When soil and water is contaminated there is no other way for things to go, than for the food supply to become contaminated.

A salmon or a dolphin cannot swim in mercury tainted waters and not consume those poisons. A shrimp cannot live in its' watery universe without being affected by sewage pumped into waterways. An apple cannot expect to grow absent of chemicals when the farmer sprays every tree with herbicides and pesticides designed to kill all. A seed, meant to grow corn, and packaged Round-Up Ready can never hope to be a clean food. It simply is not.

Being overweight, obese, underweight, undernourished and toxic are conditions leading to the same result: we are not at our optimum level of wellness.

---

1   http://www.cbc.ca/news/health/pollution-worldwide-deaths-1.4363613

IS FOOD EVEN REAL?

The purpose of food has remained the same for millennia. No one, that we know of yet, has been able to survive without eating. Everybody knows you have to eat to survive. However, what has changed dramatically is what you are eating. Food is not food anymore. At no time in the existence of man, have you been exposed to the kinds of processed and transformed substances you are eating now. The experiment with processed food, although helping you save time, did so at the cost of your health.

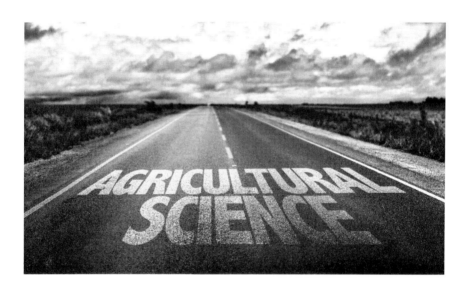

Eating anything has become a complex effort.

Foods come with ingredients on labels that read like a science experiment. No lay person understands what many of these multi-syllabic words mean. Most of them are chemicals but how do you and I really know? The truth is, you don't. Scientists, paid a rich salary by food conglomerates to "create packaged foods", are always a step ahead of you. You will never know all the tricks they are up to. We will not know, in enough time, what the repercussions are. You will never get there before they do.

You must navigate the shelves of supersized grocery stores, in a frenzied pursuit of groceries. What is on display in these mammoth food warehouses is food but food of questionable value. No longer can you buy a simple package of oats. Now oats come complete with high fructose corn syrup, the potential of containing allergenic ingredients, have been refined to the point of being devoid of nutrients, and is very likely genetically modified so much so, that it no longer resembles its' earliest cousin.

Twenty-first-century food is going to be real food.
Real food is food that is truly nourishing for the
consumer, the community, and the planet.

- Kimbal Musk

Food is no longer food. It is well for You to understand this. Food today is not the food of yesteryear. Food today is not even the food of 20 years ago. Food has been altered thanks to science, the marketplace, culture and energies we cannot begin to understand.

There is an overabundance of calories yet shockingly a lack of nutrients. You are starting to see now, particularly in the United States, some nutrient-based diseases that are reappearing. Who would ever have thought that Rickets, the English disease of the seventeenth century that was abolished after the Industrial Revolution, would be a disease making a frightening return in 2017? This is caused by a calcium, vitamin D and essential fatty acids deficiencies, nutrients we apparently forgot to be concerned about in the modern era.

NUTRIENT LACK

You are nutrient starved so it's no wonder your body is responding by becoming diseased. Bone issues like osteopenia and osteoporosis are common now thanks to poor diet[2]. Heart disease is still the number one killer, based on an over consumption of sugar - not fat as formerly thought. Cancer is also part of the growing state of diseases. One in two will experience cancer by 2020. Fertility is less readily possible for young couples. You were born with the gift of being able to create life and, even that, thanks to the diminished state of your food and state of wellness, may soon not be readily accomplished without external help. Counting calories is not a safe strategy to lose weight, as food doesn't nourish you anymore.

In the upcoming chapters, we will demystify some myths about food, notably about fat, cholesterol, carbohydrates and sugar. Your society now faces an overload of misleading information, which contributes to our confusion and malnutrition. Nowadays, everyone is "an expert". Doctors with as little as two hours of training in nutrition are trying to tell us what to eat and getting it wrong. You could get information about wellness on the back of a cereal box, in a commercial or in a glitzy fashion magazine. Everyone seems to be an expert. Who do you trust? Everywhere you turn, you are bombarded with information, but, who is right?

This book has been written through our collective wisdom to help you navigate a path to wellness. What we present are the tried and true foundations upon which to build this journey. Remember optimal wellness is your birthright. To the question "Who is right?" you will be able to answer with confidence: "I am".

---

2   www.bones.nih.gov

KEY CONCEPTS:

Obesity and illnesses have spiked over the past decades.

Food is not food.

Processed, refined and engineered foods are part of a disastrous experiment that is leaving us overweight and unhealthy.

Disease is on the rise.

We live in a world of abundance in calories and yet, we are undernourished and have developed multiple food intolerances.

Our environment is dramatically changed from what it used to be.

It has become very complicated to make educated and clean food choices.

CHAPTER 6:

WHAT IS BEING CLEAN FROM THE INSIDE OUT?

"...a state of complete physical, mental, and social well-being, and not merely the absence of disease or infirmity."

- World Health Organization

Being clean and healthy comes from within and is part of who you can be. The notion of living a clean lifestyle does need some context. We are not referring to keeping clean, as in avoiding drugs or participating in illicit behavior. What is meant by "living clean" is following a lifestyle that addresses the three components of wellness, as defined by the World Health Organization:

"...a state of complete physical, mental, and social well-being, and not merely the absence of disease or infirmity."
- The World Health Organization

If you consider the pursuit of wellness, then you know that you have to make an effort in all three of these areas in order to make a positive impact on your physical self. You can't only work out and hope you are well. You can't just Eat Clean® and think that's enough. And you can't work out and Eat Clean® and forget about your emotions. Each component is significant.

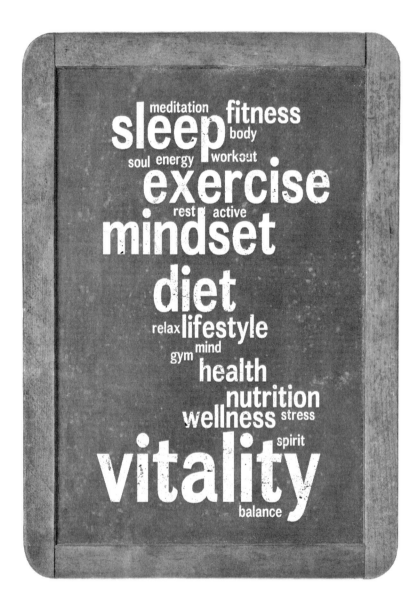

The World Health Organization, the global governing body of wellness, describes wellness as not simply being disease free. Wellness is the presence of robust practice in Eating Clean®, Exercising and Emotional Self Care. You are at your best when you practice, to the best of your ability, the three E's of wellness which work together to support a clean lifestyle, resulting in optimal wellness for you.

Eating Clean®

Exercise

Emotional Wellness

When you translate this, you see that wellness is not simply the absence of disease. It is the presence of certain lifestyle practices including Eating Clean®, Exercise and Emotional/Mental/Social agency. Wellness is never a fixed point on a line. You don't arrive at wellness one day and stop pursuing it. You are constantly changing and so is your life. You must organically pursue wellness every day. Wellness is an active process of participating in making healthy choices to support a robust life.

"Wellness is a dynamic process of change and growth." – The World Health Organization.

You cannot hope to defend against any of the above plagues if you are in a "less than" state. The body requires all organs to be in a state of homeostasis – perfect balance - in order to conduct the activities necessary to survive and thrive. Pollution, toxicity, stress, poor nutrition, lack of exercise, ignorance, lack of access to proper nourishment and apathy lead to an unclean self; a body unable to show up to do the job of living.

When you come to understand that every meal presents an opportunity to nourish yourself rather than simply fill your belly, you experience a dramatic shift in your approach to food. Hunger is meant to be satiated yes, but not with a mindlessly consumed bag of potato chips. There is exactly zero nourishment in that bag of chips. The body will cry out for nourishment until you ultimately become deaf or until you make change and believe me, the body is sending messages to you all day long.

To change the current situation, which is dangling on the precipice of disaster, you must change the way you think about food. You must change how you eat, what you eat, when you eat and why you eat. You must return to mindful eating. Eating to sustain life. Eating to thrive. Eating to nourish the body to its' fullest potential. Eating to restore the brilliance that is human life.

When you match your mindset to your eating you become clean inside and out. You align the mind, which thinks of wellness every minute, with the food that builds us to our highest level of magnificence. You clean yourself out and find that inner glow that is unmistakably wellness. That is why being clean is an inside job. Clean and healthy is not something you reach or something you possess, acquire or collect. Being clean is a feeling encompassed in vibrant energy that is impossible to ignore.

We hope, in these pages, to help you on your journey of self-discovery. The goal is to align you with your truest definition of health, not someone else's, but still acknowledging the need to be well through Eating Clean, Exercise and Emotional Self-care. Clean and healthy is less about what you do and more about how you do it and how you feel while doing it.

Being clean is achieved when you are in touch with your deeper structure. It is when you control your emotions and find alignment within yourself. Being clean is to align every layer of yourself, in order to find your life purpose. Your layers represent the base of this book and the foundation of the DNA System.

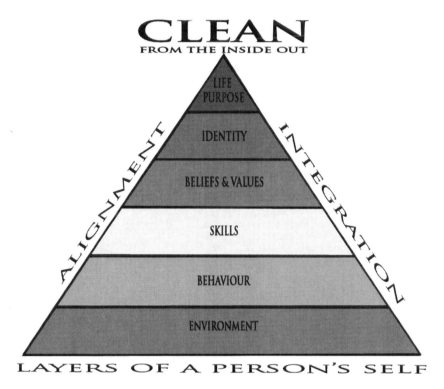

Living clean is to live in an environment that serves you, with behaviours that use and build your skills, as you follow your beliefs and values to live your full identity and reach your life purpose.

Living clean is to live in an environment that serves you, with behaviours that utilize your skills and build them, as you follow your own beliefs and values to live your full identity and reach your life purpose.

Clean living leads to a fulfilling life with the ultimate goal of reaching your personal best! You will learn much about yourself and mostly, you will learn that your personality and physical person, are not set in stone. You can become whatever you want to be.

Let's have a quick overview of specific characteristics that clean people have in common.

KEY CONCEPTS:

WHAT IS CLEAN?

When you match your mindset to your eating you become clean inside and out. You align the mind, which thinks of wellness every minute, with the food that builds you to your highest level of magnificence. You clean yourself out and find that inner glow that is unmistakably wellness.

Ultimately, clean living is achieved when you align and integrate all layers of yourself in order to achieve your life purpose.

This book is designed to take you on a journey through the neurological levels of your brain, embarking on the D.N.A. System that will carry you through each level and allow you to reach your full potential.

PART 3

OBSTACLES TO CLEAN LIVING

CHAPTER 7:

IS OUR CULTURE
MAKING US UNHEALTHY?

"Sharing food has always had a central place
in civilized societies; it's no accident that so
many of our cultural, religious and patriotic
rituals are involved with eating."

Ruth Reichl

We learn to eat at our mother's breast as infants and at the kitchen table as youngsters. Eating is a complex business, influenced not only by culture, family traditions and geography, but by what is available to us. According to Bee Wilson, in First Bite, "everything we eat after breast milk is up for grabs." Tanzanian babies eat bone marrow as their first food. In Laos, rice, pre-chewed by your mother, is your first food. And in Western cultures, baby's first food often comes from a jar.

Eating, outside of suckling at our mother's breast, is not something we are born knowing how to do. We must learn it. Over long periods of time.

As you grow, the process of feeding and eating becomes more and more complex. Much of what you learn is at the elbow of your parents. Their particular preferences and norms around eating will certainly be yours, at least until you leave the nest. These "norms" will follow us long into our adult lives, for better or for worse.

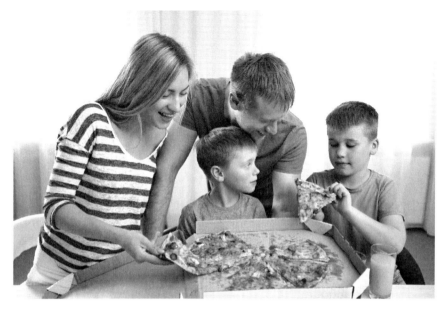

Over time, omnivorous humans have learned which foods taste good, which are delicious and which are not, which cause reactions and which may kill us. From these taste experiences you develop your tastes and preferences. The way you have eaten, up until now, has been developed as a series of learned experiences from one generation to the next. Layers of wisdom about food have accumulated to tell a narrative about what foods help you survive, or not. Your food story is a rich series of anecdotes, one layered upon the other.

Parents urge children to "finish your plate," a platitude developed from years of scarcity during war times, where leaving food on your plate was a sin because it was never clear where your next meal would come from, if at all. Although lack is still an issue for much of the world, it is easier for most of us to find food today than ever before. Almost too easy.

There are cultures that believe you must eat until you are bursting. Italians are not happy unless you have eaten enough to necessitate undoing your belt. Witness an Italian wedding where there are courses after courses and even a midnight sandwich buffet – eating goes on all night long. It is easy to see how environment shapes our beliefs about eating and how we do it. Environment has shaped your beliefs about food too.

Closer to home, when Nathalie's husband removed bread from his diet, he asked her to help him find something to replace it. He normally ate a piece of toast with his morning bowl of steel cut oats and he believed that the hot cereal wasn't enough for him to feel full. Nathalie could have helped him find something else to "replace" the bread. Instead, she helped him change the limiting belief that he needs to "feel full" after a meal.

You have plenty of room in your stomach because your ancestors needed to hunt for days before their next meal and they needed to "fill up" before their journey. In our society, where food is accessible and where you can access food anytime, anywhere, there is absolutely no need to feel full after any meal. By changing this belief, Nathalie's husband was successful at his goal and lost over twenty pounds in the process.

Your attitude towards food, including scarcity, cost, attainability, volume, quality and preparation shape every idea you have about food and thus, shape your weight, wellness and even your success outcomes.

Today's food culture however, is not so simple. You are now learning how to eat through the lens of what consumer goods companies and food scientists dictate is food. Food has become an orchestrated end product filled with various science trickery designed to seduce you into loving that particular food. Food companies hawk foods high in refined sugars, unhealthy fats, refined salt and other such taste experiences. Children learn to develop a taste for these, begetting a cycle of inventing ever more engineered foods, food addictions, illness and so on.

Food journalist Michael Moss revealed that "big food companies engineer foods with a chemically calculated "bliss point" designed to get us hooked." It seems, given the obesity epidemic, that you are indeed hooked. The solution is to not only learn what to eat and how but to learn and adopt new habits. No one ever ate more broccoli because someone said it was good for them. You have to set the example of how to nourish yourself through your own good self-care habits.

Most of what you know about food happens early in life, sitting at the table with our family. You learn that food is love. That it tastes good or not. You learn that it binds people together. You learn that certain foods are part of your culture and/or celebrations – the Inuit eat seal meat and blubber, Turkish folk eat kefir, the Dutch eat rolmops (pickled herring) and so it goes. You learn also that food can be withheld, as a form of punishment. Children quickly learn that consuming what's on their plate can make parents happy or angry.

If you are to correct the growing problems of nutrition and change your diet, you need to become educated and relearn many of your food responses. Change happens through reconditioning yourself, one meal at a time. Developing a healthy, knowledgeable relationship with food can serve as a life-saving practice, protecting each of you from the excesses of the obesogenic world of today.

There is also great diversity and even perhaps confusion about the number of meals to be consumed in a day. Getting "three squares" is considered the standard but for many this is impossible, particularly in developing countries, where even one meal a day is a blessing. Many are now pursing intermittent fasting as a means to control weight and boost immunity, the premise being that the fasting period helps burn fat rather than glucose. The "break" the body gets from intermittent fasting is considered a boon for the digestive tract and there is some suggestion that intermittent fasting protects against cancer.

This way of eating may serve some but by no means is this a universally sound diet plan for all. For the ever-growing segment of the population affected by blood sugar disorders, intermittent fasting may prove dangerous to their health. Indeed, those affected by blood sugar dis-regulation are better served to eat five or six smaller meals per day to help manage blood sugar levels, keeping them steady, as recommended by the American and Canadian Diabetes Associations. Eating Clean® supports this recommend-dation.

It is wise to remember that the governing biological principle true to each of you, is that you are all biologically unique. What serves for one does not always serve for another. This is why it is important to accept some agency over what and how often you eat.

For Tosca, her pre-diabetic condition that arose from being overweight, was healed by eating six smaller meals per day. Each meal was complete from a macronutrient standpoint – protein, carbohydrate and fats were always present. These smaller meals helped to regulate the previously erratic swings in her blood sugar levels – swings that she herself had caused through ignorance, poor eating and lack of exercise.

The philosophy of Eating Clean® comes from the early bodybuilders who practiced this in an extreme form to prepare for contests. Through Tosca's work with Robert Kennedy, she shaped the modern version of Eating Clean®, which embraces eating more healthy fats and plenty of greens. Meats, always a big part of a bodybuilding diet, are shifted to more plant-based protein options. Eating Clean® has helped millions learn to respect the patterns of hunger and satiation that are normal within a given day, thereby freeing them from the challenging question of "What shall I eat?" Eating Clean® has become a "food revolution" as coined by Dr. Oz.

"FAST" FOOD

What has also changed is the environment of how you eat. You eat on the fly. You eat fast. Your eating hygiene is poor and has nothing to do with how you used to spend hours cultivating fresh food, preparing and making meals from scratch or using traditional food preparation techniques.

We live in an obesogenic society where you can eat 24/7 while driving 120km per hour on the highway. You have access to food at all times. There is never a scarcity of places to access food on the fly.

KEY CONCEPTS:

Eating is a complicated business, influenced not only by culture, family traditions and geography but by what is available to you.

Food today is not the food of yesterday. What we used to grow we now create in laboratories.

You have access to food at all times and not necessarily food that nourishes 'feeds' you.

Most of what you know about food happens early in life, sitting at the table with your family.

We live in an obesogenic society where you can eat 24/7.

CHAPTER 8:

IS OUR BIOLOGY WORKING AGAINST US?

"Biology is the most powerful technology ever created. DNA is software, and protein is hardware, cells are factories."

- Arvind Gupta

THE ANATOMY OF APPETITE

You accuse willpower of sabotaging your dieting efforts because it's an excuse for making poor choices and easier not to blame yourself. Willpower does not help overcome hunger. That's because hunger is a biological function. Your brain will slow you down when you are hungry. A workout on an empty stomach feels difficult because your brain is telling you to slow down and re-fuel. Hunger is a powerful survival instinct.

As Doctor Mike Roizen, Chief Wellness Officer at the Cleveland Clinic explains, in the hypothalamus part of the brain, there is an area called the satiety center. That's the area where your brain processes hunger information. There are two types of players in this area. The eating chemicals driven by NPY (a protein called neuropeptide Y) and the satiety chemicals led by CART (cocaine-amphetamine-regulatory transcript). NPY decreases metabolism and increases appetite. CART stimulates the surrounding hypothalamus to increase metabolism, reduce appetite, and increase insulin to deliver energy to muscle cells rather than be stored as fat.

LEPTIN & GHRELIN

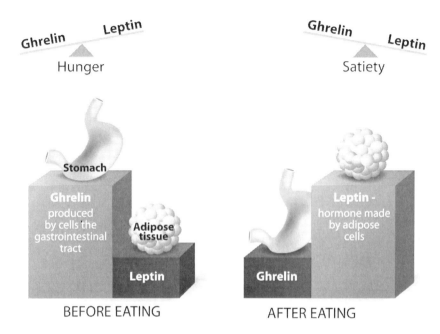

When you are hungry, NPY will slow you down. NPY will not let you use your energy because it is afraid you will run out of fuel. It slows your metabolism down. Consider that morning when you are facing a workout on an empty stomach. You feel it will be a tough workout to get through because you don't have the energy and feel weaker than normal. You hear messages like: *"I don't know what is going on, I'm doing the same workout as usual, but today is so much harder."* You then start wanting to eat. Your brain is telling you to slow down because it's in need of energy. The gas gauge light is on telling you need to refuel. NPY increases your appetite as a result.

CART has the reverse effect. When you have enough food in your stomach CART sends the brain a signal to increase your metabolism. The body is accordingly ordered to increase the level of energy. Now your brain receives a signal that the stomach is full, so it tells the body to go ahead, spend some energy, "I'm good to go, I have a full tank!" Refueled and recharged you can run and work out with energy, or you can apply yourself more fully at work. CART decreases your appetite. You need clean food in order for your brain to receive the signal that it's okay to start moving again.

WHO IS GIVING THESE SIGNALS TO THE BRAIN?

Ghrelin and leptin are the hormones responsible for sending these signals for more or less fuel to the brain. They are both stress hormones and work with NPY and CART.

Ghrelin works closely with NPY. When you have used up your fuel, ghrelin will transmit the signal to the NPY area of the brain. (Nathalie calls it the gremlin to remind herself which one is which.) Ghrelin is the little voice that tells the brain: "*I'm hungry.*" Most of you have because humans are born with this basic instinct of survival. When you are hungry, you will hear ghrelin tell you every thirty minutes, then every twenty minutes, then every fifteen, ten ... and then soon, if you still don't feed yourself, eating will be the only thing on your mind.

Leptin is the satiety hormone, or it also thought of as the hormone of energy expenditure. It will stimulate CART production. It will receive information from your stomach and notice if you are being fueled. When it perceives food in the stomach, it will give the message to the CART area of the brain to say that it's okay to move and spend energy again.

Another way ghrelin affects eating relates to sleeping patterns. When you are stressed your sleep is negatively affected. Less sleep causes chronic fatigue and increasing ghrelin levels. When you don't sleep, you gain weight.

IN LAYMAN'S TERMS

This mechanism works most efficiently with clean food. Your body is smart. Your brain is smart. We hope so because if the brain is not smart, then what is? Your body notices what you eat. Surprise! You can't just put a chocolate bar in your mouth and hope that your body will not notice. It will.

Consider that it is lunchtime. You had breakfast before work, you may even have had a snack, possibly an apple or something similar around 10:00 a.m. and now you're ready for lunch. You have not brought your lunch with you. You go to your favorite coffee shop and get a ham and cheese sandwich. It tastes alright, and you "feel" fed.

Your body has something to say about this. Your gremlin (ghrelin) is demanding food. It sees the sandwich you have just eaten and says *great*! I love ham and cheese sandwiches. But what's this? Bread. Cool! Fiber and carbs are coming. But wait a minute. Your body doesn't recognize the refined and processed white bread, so it decides to just put it aside for now and stores it—on your butt, your thighs, your stomach, anywhere it can. Meanwhile ghrelin keeps asking for food.

What about the ham? That's protein, right? But, it's processed ham, and again your body doesn't recognize it. It decides to store that too. Then there is cheese. Great! Dairy and protein together! But it's processed cheese, and your body doesn't know what this is or what to do with it. You can imagine where this ends up. The same happens with the mayo.

Ghrelin keeps asking for more and more food and will not shut up until you actually feed it. At the end of your lunch, all you've really eaten is a slice of tomato and a piece of lettuce! The limited nutrition received from these will only last a few minutes. It's no wonder you are hungry again in an hour. You haven't been fed properly.

What do you do at the end of the meal with gremlin still demanding food? You eat an oatmeal-raisin cookie. Oats should help, and a few raisins are good, but the refined sugar will be stored with the rest of the junk already accumulating around your waist. This will cause other malfunctions and slowly lead to more dire health problems.

Now keep your attention on the next few lines because we are not done here. Some of you are thinking right now that it's okay to store some garbage when you work out a lot. You think that the "stuff" you ate at lunch will be burned off at 6:00 p.m. when you hit the gym.

Here is the hard truth. With no proper fuel, when you do your workout, you crash. Your workout does not and never will fix the problems you ate.

Consider when you are hungry yourself, do you open the refrigerator door, or the garbage can to look for food? You want fresh, good food energy, right? When your body needs fuel, it looks for good fuel. It won't take the fat/garbage that it did not want in the first place. It refused it once and stored it. It will not change its mind. It will not run to the garbage at the first sign of hunger. If the glycogen stores are empty, your body will look for protein for fuel and in so doing will consume your muscles and bones. When you attempt your workout, you will feel weak because you have less muscle tissue to work with, leaving you weaker than you were before. Your muscles will shrink making you lose muscle mass, not fat. The garbage will still be inside you, but the muscles will be shrinking, changing your body composition. In turn, as muscles shrink, your metabolic rate decreases, causing more weight gain.

So how do you get rid of your garbage? You need to contract your muscles, so they get rid of the accumulated "stuff" for you. Therefore, it is critical you feed yourself properly before your workout.

A BIG DINNER BUT NOT FED

Recently Nathalie went out for dinner with her husband to an Italian restaurant. As an occasional treat, Nathalie likes pasta, and that is one of the reasons why she usually makes her own pasta so that she can control the kind of flour she uses - she grinds her own flour too. Restaurants usually use white refined flour. At that Italian restaurant, white flour was used to make the pasta. The meal tasted fantastic, however it was not real food. The appetizer was white bread dipped in extra virgin olive oil and balsamic vinegar. Yum! Then they had pasta for their meal. And as a treat, Nathalie even had some decadent chocolate.

Nathalie and her husband walked back home from the Italian restaurant absolutely stuffed. But when they got home, Nathalie made herself a nut butter cracker before bed. Her husband looked at her and said: "Are you crazy? We just ate a huge meal!"

The problem is that they had not been properly fed. The bread was white bread made with refined flour, the pasta was white pasta also made with refined white flour, and we all know there is nothing healthy in conventional chocolate cake. No component of their meal nourished her body, except the tablespoon of extra virgin olive oil. It tasted delicious, and Nathalie loved it, but she had to teach a fitness class in the morning, and she knew she couldn't do it if her body had not been fed. You have to make up for your mistakes, and that doesn't mean starving yourself because starving doesn't help. It means getting back on track to fueling your body properly. Nathalie got up the next morning and had a protein shake before her workout to make sure she had good fuel to allow her muscles to contract and activate her metabolism instead of slowing it down.

KEY CONCEPTS:

Ghrelin is the hunger hormone that works with the NPY area of your brain, telling you to eat when your stomach is empty. It slows you down to preserve energy.

Leptin is the satiety hormone working with your CART, letting you know your tank is full and allowing you to use energy.

When you are hungry, you have to feed yourself with real food, otherwise, your brain will keep asking for more until you are properly nourished.

CHAPTER 9:

IS STRESS AT CAUSE?

*"The greatest weapon against stress is our
ability to choose one thought over another."*

William James

Stress spills out as a governing response, in all aspects of our lives from performing in a marathon, to taking exams or becoming overwhelmed with the hectic pace of modern life.

Modern research shows a strong link between stress and eating behaviours. It is important to remember that stress can either make you over eat or under eat, both of which can be problematic. The numbers show there is consistent evidence that people will eat food that is higher in sugar and fat when stressed. While this type of eating might produce some short term psychological relief, the result is always an increase in abdominal obesity and cardiovascular disease.

Tosca tells us about what happens in her own life: "When I am stressed, I cannot eat. During the time that my late husband was dying from lung cancer, I was unable to follow my own good advice about eating consistently. I lost 15 pounds in a few short weeks. I didn't look or feel well. But stress has that kind of effect on me." This appears to be the opposite of most people, who tend to overeat. "Eating Clean® brought me back and I knew that if I wanted to have a decent shot at living a good life, I needed to put some nutrition back into my body". Eating Clean helped Tosca get back on track to a stronger, more sound state of wellness.

Chronic stress is also a strong indicator for weight gain, especially in men (Nutrition Volume 23, Issues 11-12, November-December 2007, Pages 887-894).   This research correlates to the sky-rocketing overweight and obesity rates in North America, if not the world. Therefore, being aware of your stress levels and finding ways to better manage your stress will be critical lifestyle skills needed to help you make changes in your eating habits, and fostering Eating Clean®.

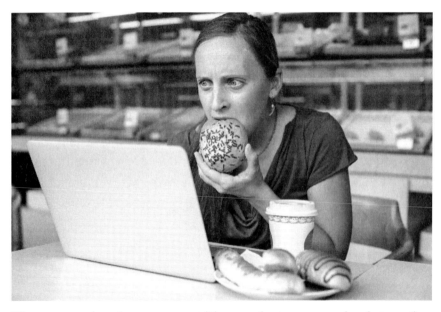

The connection between nutrition and stress can be interesting because usually making clean food choices are the last thing on your mind when you perceive stress. Instead there is a tendency to eat everything that is not good, so it's highly unlikely that nutritional deficiencies are the cause of stress, at least outwardly. But our nutritional needs do change when we are experiencing stress, so the best strategy is to help the body "cope" with stress by providing enough of the nutrients which are in greater demand or are more difficult to acquire when we are stressed. This is one compelling reason that Eating Clean® is a powerful lifestyle method of managing wellness. When we Eat Clean® we build up a powerful foundation of wellness, strength, robustness and vitality so that when a stressful event comes along, we are not plunged into illness, but we have a cushion of resilience that helps us withstand the stress.

Nathalie recalls, when she was a child, her mother always stressed the importance of having a nutritious breakfast on an important day. i.e. when she had an exam, a dance performance or later in life, an important meeting.

The following example demonstrates what we mean. The Boston Marathon is the world's oldest annual marathon and ranks as one of the world's most prestigious and challenging road racing events. Participants must qualify to be allowed to run the 26-mile course and the qualification standards are high. You must be able to run it in a respectable and fast paced 3-4 hours. It takes weeks and months, even years, of preparation. Once the race is over, 50% or more of the contestants fall ill. Doctors call the 72 hours after an endurance event the "open window" for infection.

The reason for this is that, while you are preparing for your contest, your body reacts to the regular stress from exercise in the same way it would react to an infection. Your immune system gets pumped up as you do, handling and destroying pathogens efficiently. When you become an endurance or elite athlete however, things change. The continual stress works in the opposite way, over challenging your immune system and often overwhelming it. The body is flooded with stress hormones during an intense physical event, cortisol being the primary one, and the immune system switches into defensive mode. As you cross the finish line, the protective effect provided by your immune system decreases much more quickly than the levels of your stress hormones do, thus making you susceptible to illness.

While 95% of the population is not an endurance athlete, you can relate to this and experience this phenomenon in everyday life, thanks to the hectic pace you set. After an important meeting or a build-up to an event, you tend to succumb to infection, which explains why you often get sick during the holiday season, an intensely stressful time for most. You can now understand how critical it is to keep your nutrition clean.

There are several ways stress affects weight and eating. As noted, stress causes most of you to "stress eat." Stress eating is considered emotional eating and why wouldn't it be? For many, eating is THE stress response, the one that you reach for when they've had it! Life is fast paced, sweat inducing, and hairy. When you are totally immersed in the stress response, you want a quick fix, a way to handle the beating heart and sweaty palms.

The usual "fix" is to grab something crunchy or sweet. And you are not to blame to crave such foods. Human beings are wired for sweet. The brain knows simple carbohydrates will satisfy rapidly and predictably thanks to the rush of glucose that "feeds" the brain. Such foods provide an immediate "feel good" response in the brain, however short-term it may be. Emotional response eating contributes to excess calories and when this becomes a normal response pattern, thus a habit, causes weight gain.

THE STRESS RESPONSE

Stress can be positive or negative and both are necessary. Torres & Nowson (2007) define stress as "any general physical response of the body that either overwhelms or threatens to overwhelm it and its ability to maintain homeostasis."

In general, stress happens when demands exceed our coping capabilities. The reaction to stress varies depending on what is happening in your life and your individual character. Stress is both a biological and physiological response to a perceived threat you have no resources or ability to master. The "stressor" or threat that causes stress, triggers the release of cortisol, a stress hormone designed to shut down non-essential functions and give you bursts of energy in the event of a lion, tiger or bear! Unfortunately, modern life provides plenty of opportunities for increased stress and very little opportunity for relaxation and calm. Therefore, our stress responses are hyper-stimulated, with little or no reprieve. Your body is under routine assault by metabolic processes intended to be life-saving, that ironically now contribute to the increase of disease and death in this culture.

This is one of the reasons why relaxing times, enjoying a meal with family and friends, yoga classes, exercise and meditation are so crucial to overall health, as well as clean living. Creativity is also halted when the brain shifts into "fight or flight" mode. The antidote that will create balance, health, and ultimately clean living, is a conscious approach to mitigating the stress response and creating a supportive environment for ourselves.

If you look at it as a trigger for balance-seeking state, then you can use stress to your advantage and use it as an opportunity for growth. If you do not have what it takes to deal with the situation, you will build it, learn and grow. The D.N.A. System will teach you how to respond to stress, so you can access the wisdom of what used to be a well-kept secret to a select few.

PRESSURE VS. STRESS

What is the difference between pressure and stress?

Pressure is external. It is what happens to you in your life. It surrounds you every day. It is your alarm clock not going off and making you late, it is traffic, it is running out of milk, our boss holding us accountable for extra work, our child not feeling well, an unexpected expense, one of our parents falling ill and so on. External pressure and its' negative effects are presented to you every day.

This external pressure creates stress in your body. Stress is internal. A good way to get rid of stress is to take time for yourself and focus, meditate or have a good sweat! Any type of exercise will help you clear away the stress, momentarily. Yes, the external pressure will still be there, but it will not affect you for the time being. You will feel like a million dollars after you exercise and say to the external pressure: "Bring it on!" Later on, we will show you how to make this temporary stress-free state of mind last. You will learn how to let go of the built-up negative emotions that are at the root of your response to external pressure.

Stress impacts your health. It can be the element that keeps you from reaching your goals or not. Stress is what you create in your body when you face external pressure. It is not all toxicity and negativity. It is what you choose to do with it. Athletes intentionally put themselves through stress and stressful situations to adequately prepare for races. The best grapes in the world often grow in the most challenging soils and conditions where the grape vine has learned to make the most of it.

Negative emotions like anger, fear or hurt result from challenging experiences. They are not designed to bring you down. They provide the additional boost of adrenaline you need to pay attention to what you are facing so that you can step up your game and get to the next level in your life. The stress caused by these emotions is used as a stepping-stone to grow.

Let's have a closer look at the brain and how the different parts of your brain work for or against you.

KEY CONCEPTS:

STRESS RESPONSE

Making clean food choices are the last thing on your mind when you perceive stress.

Stress is experienced when a "stressor" is applied to your life and you feel you don't have the resources to respond. The key is to trust that everything that happens to you would not occur if you did not have the tools to deal with it. If not, that means the stressor (or external pressure) is happening for you to grow and build the tools you need.

PRESSURE vs STRESS

Pressure represents the external reasons why you create stress inside your body.

Stress impacts your health. You need to recognize external pressure as growth opportunities.

PART 4

THE FOUNDATIONAL LAYERS OF THE THINK Yourself® D.N.A. SYSTEM

CHAPTER 10:

CLEAN LIVING COMES FROM WITHIN

"Whatever we plant in our subconscious mind
and nourish with repetition and emotion will
one day become a reality."

Earl Nightingale

Your brain is among the most complex structures on earth. Asleep or awake it controls every moment, movement and thought. Think about it: Do you have to tell yourself to breathe? To swallow? To blink? Remind your hair to grow? Your brain controls it all without you having to think about it. The brain is wondrous!

THE LOGICAL MIND

You use your logical mind on the surface in your day-to-day activities. Your logical mind is the voice you hear in your head. The one you use to make decisions. You give your logical mind vast responsibilities, paired with hope, as to the extent of its power. The logical mind can process an average of between five and nine pieces of information simultaneously. While you are reading this book, you are likely also able to notice an average of seven other things.

For example, as you read, you can picture yourself understanding these concepts; you can see yourself in your little black dress you haven't been able to wear for a while, you can see what is on your desk, hear if there is music playing in the background, notice that your pants feel uncomfortable and so on. You can do all of these things at the same time. Doesn't that sound magical? Your logical mind is powerful. Just wait until you hear about the best part of your brain. The logical mind is actually quite restricted. Have you ever noticed when you are driving to a new address, as you come closer and start looking at civic numbers on the doors, you need to lower the volume of the radio in your car? The five to nine pieces of information juggled by your logical mind get filled up very quickly. As you are driving, with the foot on the break/accelerator, noticing the red light ahead, the child about to cross the street and the handsome guy in the car next to yours all at the same time, makes listening to "the music" that one more piece of information your brain can't process. It becomes an overwhelming task.

When you are not overloaded with external thoughts about what you are doing, you also generate thoughts with your logical mind. According to the research of Dr Raj Rahunathan Ph.D., the brain generates between 12,000 and 50,000 thoughts per day. Unfortunately, up to 70% of these thoughts are negative. With that many negative thoughts you wonder what is wrong with you? Why is everybody else successful except you? You question why you haven't been chosen and tell yourself you are probably not good enough. You think you would have time to focus on your own health if you didn't have to take care of everyone else. You think everyone is better and knows more than you. These negative thoughts, either looking for approval or control, or demonstrating feelings of inferiority, represent most of your daily internal dialogue.

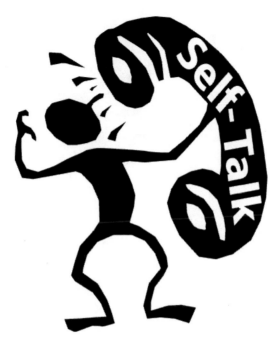

When you start paying attention to everything you tell yourself, you realize why your efforts for success at clean living have been in vain.

> *"Would you want to be your friend if you talked to them the same way you talk to yourself?" - Unknown*

It is possible your logic might not be so logical. And all these years, you relied on it solely for the most important decisions in your life. The good news is that the voices inside your head have volume controls. You can make them louder, you can make them softer, you can make them say what you want and in whatever tone of voice. You will learn about this in the NEW YOU and ACTUALIZE sections of this book. For now, let's have a look at another part of your mind.

THE UNCONSCIOUS MIND

While the logical mind is busy talking down to you, the unconscious mind is busy working, understanding everything, down in the deep structure of yourself. The unconscious mind can handle over two million pieces of information every second, (while our little logical mind was only able to handle seven, on average). Everything you have seen, done, thought, heard and felt is organized in your deeper structure waiting for your recall. Your unconscious mind sees everything. It reads every sign and all advertisements while you drive to work. It hears every conversation around you, whether you are paying attention or not. It feels all the non-verbal signs that others are communicating to you without your knowledge. It captures all the "behind-the-scenes" details that the logical mind misses. It takes every piece of information and deletes, distorts and filters everything to create your model of reality.

Your unconscious mind has so much information it is dying to share with you. The problem is that you are not trained to think with your unconscious mind. Before today, you might even have thought that the unconscious mind was a one-way drawer. You may have thought that the logical mind is the one used for thinking and that the unconscious mind is the one used for storing.

Have you ever lost something that you had in your hand minutes before? You know you put it somewhere. You start thinking with your logical mind and wonder where you put it? Where can it be? You had it just now. Where did it go? The reason you can't seem to find it is because you are asking the wrong part of your brain. Your logical mind was probably busy with six other things and did not notice what you did with it. You want to ask your unconscious mind where the missing item went. It knows. Always. After all, it was you that put it somewhere. You are not asking your unconscious mind to read somebody else's mind. Just yours.

RELAX AND ASK YOUR UNCONSCIOUS MIND

Numerous pages could be devoted to sharing the stories of your life and how your unconscious mind helped you find something, because you are constantly using your unconscious mind to find things.

Tosca describes an example of such a story. "As a writer, I depend on stories as a way to share my expertise. The best way to share knowledge and educate others is through story. I wanted to tell the story of the numerous difficult events that happened to me over the past several years. This started with the sudden death of my stepson and was quickly followed by the death of my husband, my true love, one year later in 2012. Soon after I discovered that Robert's publishing business, that had put out ground breaking magazines like MuscleMag, Clean Eating and Oxygen, had been insolvent, forcing me to declare bankruptcy in 2013. This was then followed by the discovery that Robert had left no monies or life insurance dollars for the family. I was thrown into financial disaster and couldn't find a way to make sense of any of it let alone tell my story. And yet the writer in me wanted to tell it. I simply couldn't find a way to do it. Until, six years later, while travelling home on a plane and after having meditated for an hour, I received a message (from the Universe). The message said: DO NOT WRITE A BOOK ABOUT YOUR TROUBLES. WRITE A BOOK ABOUT YOUR LEARNINGS. THAT IS HOW YOU CAN BEST HELP PEOPLE. And so, I began to write. When I let my subconscious mind solve the problem for me, I received guidance and solutions. Now I can write again!

Here is one story that happened to Nathalie as she had misplaced her driver's license. Somehow, it was not in its' usual slot in her wallet anymore, and she could not figure out where she had left it. She went to bed that night, incapable of sleeping, going through every possibility in her head. She finally stopped the wheel-spinning process happening in her head. She asked her unconscious mind to do the thinking for her while she fell asleep. As Nathalie slept she tasked her unconscious mind to find her driver's license and to tell her where it was the following morning.

When she got up, after a long restful night, she did not remember that she had been worried about her drivers' license the night before. On the other hand, she remembered that she had to scan a document that needed to be sent to her financial advisor. She went straight to her office, signed the document and lifted the cover of the scanner to scan the document. Sure enough, there was her driver's license, on the scanning platform. She thanked her unconscious mind that had found a way, through the financial document reminder, to let her know where to find it.

Using the D.N.A. System, you can make your logical mind and unconscious mind communicate so that you have access to that deeper structure, where everything is clear and simple. The answers are all within you, waiting to be accessed.

In Tosca's example, Tosca struggled to make sense of the challenges she faced and how to tell her story. Initially her response was to react negatively. It took some time to find a new path, a new way to respond and when she did, she received numerous gifts, changing her perspective about her challenging years completely.

In her example, Nathalie could have let stress and panic get in the way and continue to worry about losing her drivers' license. She did for a few minutes. It is not that Nathalie or Tosca never go back to reacting. That still happens. The difference is that they are aware it is happening, notice and it and make a choice not to remain in reactive mode for long.

With practice, you get used to exploiting the power of your unconscious mind. When the many layers of negative emotions and thoughts have been removed, there is a clear path between your logical and unconscious mind. The NEW YOU part of this book, the N of the D.N.A. System, will allow you to remove the junk from the drawer so you can access the amazing YOU at the bottom of it. This communication with your deeper structure is one of the most powerful techniques you will learn, one that liberates you from the grip of your negative past.

The power hidden in the words you use every day is underrated. You will see in this book how you can use the power of words to serve you in achieving your goals. What's in this book for you? Power to think for yourself. We will not give you advice and tell you what to do. We will show you how to generate the solution yourself. You need to make your own decisions in order to stick with the consequences. Your own brain needs to generate ideas. So we, the authors, don't give advice. We will suggest clean solutions and it will be up to you to adapt them to your own model of reality. This book is not about us. It is about YOU. You will find your own answers. We will ask powerful questions and help your unconscious mind deliver the answers that will serve you best.

Have you ever told something to someone numerous times only to find, months later they have the brilliant idea of doing what you had been suggesting? You want to shake them and say: "Well, that is what I have been telling you to do for months!!!" But they were not listening. They have to be the ones getting the idea themselves. When you told them, at the time, their brain was not ready to process that information. Unless they generate the idea themselves, you can tell them all you want, but it isn't going to work.

Clients and friends often ask Nathalie for advice, or they want her opinion on something. The on-going response is always: "It doesn't matter what I think. It doesn't matter what anybody thinks. I was not there. I don't know all the details about this. I don't have your background, your experiences or your values. Why don't you ask someone that was there all your life; who noticed everything; who heard every conversation and even picked up on all of the non-verbal information not picked up by anyone else? Ask your unconscious mind. It knows exactly what to do. You are very resourceful, I trust that you will figure it out."

The best moment to ask your unconscious mind a question is at night before you go to sleep. When you get into bed tonight, intentionally ask your unconscious mind to recall every piece of information you have on the subject and to give you a clear vision the next morning. It is important to ask your unconscious mind to do this WHILE YOU ARE PROFOUNDLY ASLEEP. (Otherwise, it could keep you up all night). You must specify that while your logical mind is recharging and getting long hours of rejuvenating sleep, you want your unconscious mind to work in the background and give you answers to your pressing questions in the morning.

Nathalie often uses this technique when she knows she has a writing deadline or a specific task: ''I ask my unconscious mind to write the piece overnight so that when I wake up in the morning, the words flow easily and effortlessly. I even use my unconscious mind to pack before a trip. It knows every single piece of clothing I own, it knows which ones I prefer, which ones are the most comfortable and appropriate for the trip". Some people say that it can even tell the future and that your unconscious mind knows if it is going to be sunny or cold. So let your unconscious mind do the packing for you. "Usually, the morning after asking my unconscious mind to make the packing list for me, I only need 15 minutes and my suitcase is closed!"

Imagine how fabulous your life will be when you can access all the knowledge and the experience your unconscious mind has for you! You always have all the answers to your problems within you and you are about to learn how to access it.

PEOPLE HAVE ALL THE RESOURCES THEY NEED TO SUCCEED.

You already possess every resource you need to succeed. This opens up vast possibilities. By resources, we mean the internal responses and external behaviours needed to achieve a desired response. Often you have resources you haven't considered. Maybe you know someone who shows good leadership skills at work but can't manage his or her children. You may be wondering why you can be so polite with strangers and yet, be abrupt when it comes to talking to you spouse or partner. Why is it that you can have a skill - patience for example - and not use it? If you have the skill, you have it. It is like being pregnant. You cannot be a little bit pregnant. You are or you aren't. When you have a skill, you have it. It is there in your belly. Period. So if you can be patient with strangers, you can be patient with your partner. It is just a matter of re-wiring your brain.

All that you need to succeed is within you and is waiting to be discovered. Stop limiting yourself. You already have the internal brainpower and the capability if you choose to apply your mind. You don't have to wait…. you don't have to say, "When I get this, then I will do that." You have all the tools in your brain right now. You can be whomever you choose to be today. You don't need to read another book on clean living. You will not have to search for the magic pill that will provide you with your ideal weight or optimal health. You have everything you need within you now to achieve success. When you follow this principle, you will trust that your unconscious mind will guide you to find the tools and present to you everything you need.

Keep your eyes open and trust your unconscious mind to show you everything. Trust that your powerful unconscious mind will ensure that you are introduced to the right people, the right material, the right ideas to make success unfold. When you set your unconscious mind on a mission, it keeps working for you in the background as you continue to live your life. It makes sure that things happen well for you. You will see in the next chapter how you can use your unconscious mind like you would use a personal assistant.

KEY CONCEPTS:

The logical mind can only handle 5 to 9 things at a time while the unconscious mind can manage over 2 million pieces of information per second.

You tend to only ask input from your logical mind, which is negative 70% of the time.

You don't tend to implement other people's advice. You need to generate the solution themselves.

Ask your unconscious mind for answers. Answers reside inside you in your deeper structure, which can be accessed once all the negative emotions have been cleared.

WE HAVE ALL WE NEED

You have all the resources you need to succeed. You can stop looking for external solutions to your problems. It is all there waiting for you inside.

If you want advice, don't ask around. Ask yourself.

CHAPTER 11:

YOUR PERSONAL ASSISTANT

*"I believe that you will not get what you want
unless you ask for it."*

Nia Vardalos

Your unconscious mind can be used as a personal assistant. Whatever you tell your brain, it will happen. It is like writing software for your brain. You can decide what you want to be and have that written on the software. It is like re-inventing yourself. What are you going to be?

PLACE YOUR ORDER

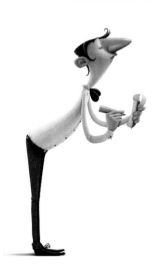

Your personal assistant inside your head takes notes and makes sure that everything you say or think gets done. It's like having a waiter in your head, standing ready with a note pad to take your order and then running to the kitchen to place it. Whatever you think or say will get cooked by the chef and brought back to you exactly as you ordered it. You must be careful when you think and when you talk, your personal assistant is always listening. If you wake up in the morning and look at yourself in the mirror and say: "Oh, my! I look horrible! I look tired!" Your personal assistant writes that on the list: "Got it: look terrible & tired, I will make that happen." You continue with your day saying to yourself that you feel stupid, or inadequate, or you don't want to be stressed and you hate rushing everywhere. Your personal assistant adds 'stupid', 'inadequate', 'stressed' and 'rushing' to the list. You let the voice inside your head tell you that you are a failure and a fraud. 'Failure' and 'Fraud' get added to the list. You tell yourself to not forget this (maybe a folder you are supposed to bring to the office). You show up at the office without the folder that you had 'programmed' yourself to 'forget'. All your brain can hear is: Horrible, Tired, Stupid, Inadequate, Stress, Rush, Failure, Fraud, Forget the folder.

Close your eyes for a moment and do NOT visualize Mickey Mouse wearing a yellow tuxedo standing on top of an elephant, did you see him? Of course, you did. Even if we said: "Do Not visualize Mickey Mouse...." Your brain doesn't process negation. You must be careful! People sit in Nathalie's office all the time telling her they don't want to be stressed anymore, they don't want to be fat, they don't want to be impatient with their kids and they don't want to be rushing all the time! It is as if they are telling their contractor that they want him/her to paint the kitchen *not* blue. Your contractor won't know what color you want your kitchen to be if you only use the colors you don't want. What do you want instead? Use your brain wisely, think and say what you want, not what you don't want!

We often hear people say, "I wish I liked healthy food." Who told you that you don't like that? You did!! You can write fresh software for your brain. Have you heard people say: "I am very bad with names." The answer is always the same: Why aren't you? Who decided that you were bad with names? Who made the call?

You may say: "I am a morning person" or "I am a night owl." You have conditioned yourself to be that way and you believe it. Nathalie says on the subject: '' If I need to stay up late, then I am an evening person and if I need to get up early, then I tell myself that I am a morning person. I can be both. Whatever is serving me." If a thought is not serving you, change it! Just start believing you are good at remembering names. There is so much room in your brain, you can remember multiple things you don't need, so why wouldn't there be room for a few extra names?

The brain is supremely powerful, more so than the most powerful computer. If you think you can, *you can*. You grew up with different patterns and you've been told these patterns for 20, 40 or more years. The good news is that you can rewrite these patterns. If you tell your brain you are willing to learn how it feels to live Clean, it will make you stop wasting time on non-important tasks. It will teach you how to master the skills you need to reach your goals. Use caution when talking to your brain.

THE CHEF KNOWS HOW TO COOK

Sometimes, you undervalue your worth. You feel that you have to restrain your demands to what you know. You don't allow yourself to dream because you don't know exactly how to get there. Let's go back to the example of the waiter awaiting your order at the restaurant. When you order something from the waiter, you don't necessarily need to know how to cook the dish you have ordered. You just place your order. It doesn't matter if you know how to prepare the dish you want. The chef placed the dish on the menu, making it clear the chef knows how to prepare it. The chef is like your unconscious mind. It knows exactly how to make your "order" happen. If you were able to dream it, it means that your chef knows how to cook it. You would not have been able to dream it if you did not have what it takes to realize it. All you have to do is to place your order with the "waiter" in your unconscious mind. The waiter will run to the kitchen and bring back your meal. When you are clear with what you want and what you expect from your unconscious mind, it starts working for you in the background while you continue to live your life. Your chef gathers all the ingredients for your "dish." You will then be guided into being at the right place at the right time. It whispers answers to your ears when you are about to learn something that will generate results towards your goal. Trust that you have everything you need inside. You got this! Just place your order!

Now that you know more about the brain, let's find out about the components of the brain responsible for your programming.

KEY CONCEPTS:

YOUR PERSONAL ASSISTANT

Your brain executes whatever you input into your software. All you have to do is dream and place your order to your unconscious mind.

If you can dream of something, it means that your chef knows how to make it happen.

CHAPTER 12:

NEURAL PATHWAYS

"A single footstep will not make a path on the earth, so a single thought will not make a pathway in the mind. To make a deep physical path, we walk again and again. To make a deep mental path, we must think over and over the kind of thoughts we wish to dominate our lives."

– Henry David Thoreau

So far, you have learned that your food, your culture and the way you live in society are, in part, responsible for interfering with your ability to live clean. You have also learned about the astonishing power of your mind, which controls everything happening to you. You will now connect the brain and how you have unintentionally programmed yourself for self-sabotage. It is revealing to know that you are responsible for whether or not you are happy with your life. The good news is that, if life is not going the way you want, it is not your fault. You have unconsciously developed negative neural pathways in your brain and you have reinforced them every time you tried something that didn't work. Then you blame yourself and feel badly. You can change this negative patterning now.

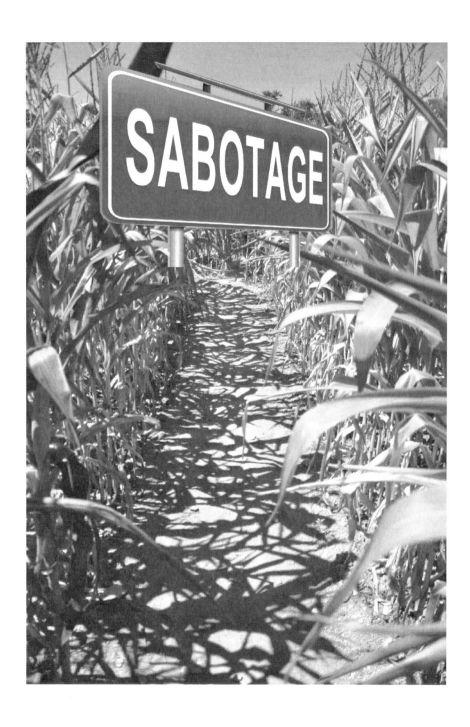

Neural pathways in your brain are responsible for your self-sabotage. Imagine you live in a house surrounded by a thick cornfield. When you leave your house, there is no other path to follow except walking on the corn. You start stepping on it, and as you walk through the field, the corn bounces back up behind you. The second time you step on the same path, the corn bounces back up, but it breaks a little and doesn't bounce back up completely. The third time, the corn is weakened even more, and so on, until, one day, you have a perfectly flat path in front of your house that leads to your preferred destination.

At this moment, when thinking about eating clean, the only path you currently know, leads to self-doubt and fear. As you continue to use your linguistic skills to change your thoughts, you will create new neural pathways inside your brain. That is how habits are built. You will begin stepping onto a new path. This may feel foreign and challenging in the beginning, as you have to "break the corn" to create the path, but once it's created and you have been there several times, the path will be clear and wide. The old path will still be there, however and there will be times you are tempted to take it. You will use the strategies you are learning in this book to stay on the new path. With time, the old path will grow new corn and will not exist as a path anymore, and you will soon forget about the old route.

The pathway you have created carries information travelling along the neurons (nerve cells) of the brain. This affects your memory. The more you review your pathways in your mind, good or bad, the more deeply they are etched in your neural pathways.

Repetition. Repetition. Repetition.

Do you remember when you switched to your mobile phone? You

had to learn a whole new way of phoning, texting, emailing, posting on social media . . . How about switching from a keyboard to a touch screen? You have learned how to use your new device and are now able to easily use your phone. This was happening while you were trying to make your new phone work for you. You likely also never had the intention of returning to your flip-phone. You knew you would be able to learn how to use your new one. Do you know any infant, attempting their first step and falling repetitively, that ever said: "Oh well, that's too hard, it's not for me, I will simply crawl my life away."

Success starts by *expecting* that you will be successful. Your chances of living a clean life rely on what you expect to happen. Let us introduce you to the notion of the *placebo effect*.

We will use the example of knee surgery. There has been diverse research conducted in Finland, Texas and Canada on knee surgery.[3]

There were two groups of people who had knee problems. In Group 1, surgery was performed on the patient and the knee was repaired. In Group 2, no surgery was performed but the patients did receive a surgical scar. Patients in Group 2 were **not** told that they were not receiving surgery. The patients in Group 2 thought that **they had** received knee surgery. Surprisingly both groups reported less pain and more mobility with their knee, regardless of whether or not they actually received surgery.

This is a demonstration of the *placebo effect*. Medicine describes the placebo effect as "a favorable response to a medical intervention — a pill, a procedure, a counseling session, you name it — that doesn't have a direct physiological effect."[4]

---

3   http://articles.mercola.com/sites/articles/archive/2014/02/07/arthroscopic-knee-surgery.aspx
4   http://www.health.harvard.edu/mind-and-mood/putting-the-placebo-effect-to-work

That change can be from spontaneous improvement, misdiagnosis, classic conditioning or subject expectancy. The power of expectancy is a favourable response to a medical intervention that doesn't have a direct physiological effect (i.e. a pill, a procedure, a counseling session).[5]

It sounds very easy doesn't it? It *is* that simple! None of these patients had received extensive training on how to re-program their brains or how to create new neural pathways when it comes to pain. But they were told to expect a different sensation when faced with the movement that used to cause them pain.

The processes and activities, coming up later in this book, contribute to recreating healthy neural pathways. The best way to heal yourself, or, going back to the subject of this book, to live a clean life, is to *expect* that it will work. Use the placebo effect to your advantage and tell yourself that you are destined to live a clean life. Whether you THINK it is doable or not… you are right.

You unconsciously create new neural pathways all the time. Every time you choose a new habit and stick to it for a while, a new neural pathway is created. You will see how this works in a few chapters when you learn how to move from *conscious incompetence* to *unconscious competence*.

Perhaps you have tried every diet on the planet; you may have been healthy for a while and then lost your way. Why? Because you think of clean living as something you will achieve at the end. You think that it is a destination. You believe that what you have to do to be healthy is 'temporary'. You think that you can give a big push right now because it is only for a short period of time. Then once you are healthy, you won't need to work as hard. You also think these

---

5   http://www.health.harvard.edu/mind-and-mood/putting-the-placebo-effect-to-work

measures you are putting yourself under are not sustainable. You believe clean living is impossible for you, and so, before you know it, you find yourself giving up and you're back to old poor habits.

None of your patterns happened overnight. If you usually take sugar in your coffee, leave it out for about two months and you'll create a new neural pathway – a new habit - in which you will enjoy your coffee without sugar. *Habit* is the key word. You want your success to be a habit, an everyday occurrence, and not an extreme, temporary measure. You see that the behaviours necessary for success are temporary, and yet, if you want something that will last, that becomes a new behaviour without effort.

AFFIRMATIONS

Affirmations in New Thought and New Age practice, refer to the practice of positive thinking and self-empowerment. This helps you foster the belief that a positive mental attitude will help you achieve success. It is becoming common practice today to use affirmations in to get achieve our goals. Affirmations can be very powerful if correctly phrased. Affirmations become the thoughts that create your reality.

Example:

"I am the architect of my well-being; I build its foundation and choose its contents, including Eating Clean®, Exercise and Emotional Selfcare."

When implementing a new habit, you must pretend it *is* a habit until it *becomes* a habit. This takes 66 days. Pretend that you want to be better at planning your meals in advance. If you tell yourself: "I am good at planning meals", the little voice inside your head may say: "Yeah, right, not at all". Use progressive statements like: ''I am willing to learn how it feels and what to do to be a good meal planner.'' When the statement feels right and true, you have found what you need to repeat in order to make it happen. Finding the statement that you believe in and repeating it until your new neural pathways are created is the key. You choose, you decide. Change the way you think about clean living. Change the way you think about food. Change the way you think about exercise. Change the way you think about emotions. The key is to find the affirmation that aligns with you when you say it out loud.

Let's look a little closer at self-sabotage.

KEY CONCEPTS:

NEURAL PATHWAYS

Your brain executes commands, as it is told how to respond, and reproduces the same response over and over until it is being taught a new path.

Your life experiences create automatic responses in your head.

These automatic responses become habits.

You get what you expect will happen.

CHAPTER 13:

SELF-SABOTAGE

"Our intention creates our reality"

- Wayne Dyer

Neural pathways are responsible for your self-sabotage. There are a few components of self-sabotage covered in this chapter.

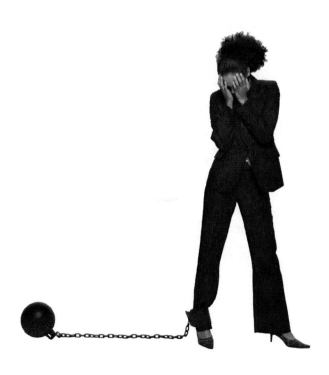

CORE VALUES & INTENTION
BEHIND THE BEHAVIOUR

The first component to consider is the *intention* behind the behaviour. You initially practice self-sabotage in order to keep safe and in your comfort zone. Most behaviours start with good intentions. Consider the teenager who takes up smoking to "belong" or the criminal who wants to "help" someone by stealing. They usually start out with good intentions, and then go downhill from there.

Finding the intention behind the behaviour becomes relevant when it comes to getting rid of a bad habit. A man who wanted to quit smoking had decreased his habit to one cigarette per day, but, was unable to completely quit. It turned out— after asking the right questions during coaching sessions—that he had not yet accepted the fact that his father had passed away. His father was a smoker, so the cigarette was connecting him with memories of his father. He did not want to let his father go. Finding the intention behind the unwanted behaviour helps to find other ways to fulfill that positive intention. Now, instead of having his one cigarette at night (the unwanted behaviour), he takes out the photo album and looks at photos of his father, so he can connect with and honour his memory. He has been smoke-free for almost 8 years and is now running half-marathons.

Your cravings are often connected to deeper memories and triggered by your senses. Consider that certain smells remind you of certain things. Mom's cooking always made you feel good. Have you ever walked into a movie theatre or a bakery? You can smell the popcorn or the freshly baked goods, and immediately the cravings start. Find the reason behind the craving and then find a different way to fulfill that craving. If you miss your mom, call her or look at some pictures. You don't need to eat a whole chocolate cake because it makes you think about her. You can still think about her and love her without having to sabotage your health!

At a very young age, you may have been taught, unconsciously, how to create emotional connections with food. Imagine that you are in a public place with your mom and you are two years old. You are in a feisty mood. You are screeching so loudly you can be heard miles away. Your mom has tried every trick, and nothing seems to be working. She has reached her tolerance limit and so have the people around, trying to ignore the scene you are causing yet staring at your mom with a condescending look, expecting her to fix this. She reverts to the last trick she knows will work. She promises you that if you stop screaming, you will be rewarded by an ice-cream. The promise of that delicious treat is enough to make you feel better. The same happened when, coming home from school at seven years old, devastated by the fact that some kids had made fun of you at school, your dad took you out for ice cream to make you feel better. Again, at twelve years old, when your sports team lost their sixth game in a row, your parents took you for ice cream to make you feel better.

Years later, it is no wonder that whenever you feel angry, hurt, disappointed or sad, you reach for food to comfort you. Your parents are not bad people. They probably got the same treatment from their parents. They did not know they were causing potential harm. Their actions came from a loving place, and they were doing their best to make you feel better.

Here is another example demonstrating how finding the intention behind the behaviour can help modify the behaviour. Nathalie had a client once who moved to a new city. Out of the blue, she kept buying a certain type of chocolate bar and devouring it, and she couldn't understand why. Every day she needed that chocolate bar. She never used to like chocolate and it was never a problem before, even when she actually worked for the manufacturer of that particular chocolate bar. (which was quite ironic, a chocolate sales rep who doesn't like chocolate).

Why was she all of a sudden eating chocolate? What had changed? She called Nathalie and said: "Nathalie, you have to help me, I am eating chocolate every day and I am going out of my mind! I never used to like chocolate! What is going on?" After a few sessions, Nathalie's client realized she missed the life she had working for the chocolate company. She had moved and was now alone in a new city. Eating chocolate was her way of coping with feeling lonely and missing her friends. She didn't really want the chocolate bar; she wanted to be with her old friends. Now, instead of eating chocolate bars, she phones or connects with her friends on email or social medias, which is a much less calorific way to fulfill the intention behind her behaviour. She has gotten back to her healthy eating habits and now lives in Australia. She still keeps in touch with her friends on the web.

In order to discover the reason behind your negative behaviours, you want to ask yourself how that negative behaviour serves you. Here is an example of Nathalie working with a client:

> What does it do for you when you eat a piece of chocolate cake?
>
> *It tastes really good and it feels like I am allowing myself a treat.*
>
> What does it do for you to feel that you are allowing yourself a treat?
>
> *It makes me feel like I am deserving of something that tastes good.*

What does it do for you to feel like you are deserving of something that tastes good?

It makes me feel like I am not depriving myself for everyone else.

So, what do you want instead of depriving yourself?

I want to take care of myself.

And what does it do for you to take care of yourself?

It makes me feel like I am worthy.

And what does it do for you to feel worthy?

It makes me feel like when I am taking care of myself first, I show self-love and then I can take care of my family because I am happier.

You have discovered that your ultimate goal is to feel that you are taking care of yourself, and NOT the piece of cake. Is there any other way you can feel that you are "treating" yourself and take care of yourself that doesn't involve something that is in fact contradictory to "taking care of yourself"?

I guess it makes no sense. What I want is to take care of myself so that I can feel happy and every time I eat cake, it makes me feel ill, guilty and crappy. At the end of the day, I am undermining my health. I guess instead I can find something else that will be healthier and will really be "taking care of myself" instead of ruining my health.

In this example, the reason why this person would eat cake is because she ultimately wanted to feel worthy and happy, so she could take care of her loved ones. Next time she gets a craving, she will remember that what she really wants is to be happy and she is aiming to make herself feel better and be her best for people around her, which is what is important to her. If family comes up in the process, it means it is really important to her. The thought of her family will give her permission to spend two hours at the gym, go for a walk, or sit and read a book with an herbal tea, without any guilt because she knows that when she does any of these things, she can be even better for her family after having taken care of herself.

You have core values, which are the things most important to you. Often, trying to align with these core values can be the root of self-sabotage. When you are aware of it and can identify your core values, you can turn the situation around and make the core values the cure instead of the cause. Honesty, Family, Freedom, Respect, Certainty, Growth and so on, could be the values that take you out of self-sabotage.

Now it's your turn. Take a few moments to reflect on a bad habit you would like to change.

''What does that do for you?'' If your bad habit had a high intention for you, a high purpose, what would that be?

_____

And then, use the answer to the question. What does that new answer do for you? What is its highest intention for you?

_____

You can also use the following question if you go backward: (if something negative comes up) ''What do you want instead?

Keep going with each answer until you find something that lights up in your head, until you tell yourself: '' That's it!!! I get it!!!''

Keep going with each answer until you find something that lights up in your head, until you tell yourself: '' That's it!!! I get it!!!''

CUMULATIVE EXPERIENCES CAUSING SELF-SABOTAGE

The second component of self-sabotage to consider is, how and why you continue to reinforce the self-sabotaging behaviour.

"There is no failure, only feedback."
- NLP Presupposition

Every action you take generates a result, whether it is a successful result or not. You hope it's a positive one but it may or may not work. Or it will work for a while and you may lose your desire for Eating Clean® for a time. Your past experience is there to teach you what did not work so that you can try something else. If nothing changes, then nothing changes.

Tosca was working with a client who is 54 years of age and who has spent three decades "trying to lose weight". Every diet she tried was met with failure. She became angry and blamed those who tried to help her as well as the diet, saying they were crap. One day, during a coaching session, she began to cry. She hoped that Tosca could fix her problem. Tosca asked her what it was she wanted in life. At that moment, she was ready to be ready to be ready to make change. She had to face a very painful truth that she wanted to leave her then husband, because he was the source of all her pain. She believed him when he called her fat, unworthy and disgusting. Because she believed it, she became it. With that revelation, she realized she had given him too much power. Over time and coaching, she took her power back and learned to love herself. She made it clear to her husband that he needed to love her for her but that she was going to love herself regardless. She lost forty-five pounds and found herself. It remains to be seen whether the husband is still on the scene or not.

If your previous attempts at clean living didn't work, then you need to receive feedback about why. Ask yourself what worked and what didn't work. Each action will give you a result. Healthy or not, whatever you do, you will obtain a result. Every action will give you information. This result will teach you a great deal about the action you performed. Was it successful? Did it work? Did it last? What can you do differently now to generate a different result? What are you missing? Is there something unrelated to dieting or food that could be affecting your health?

Everybody we meet, every article or blog we read, every action we do, come to us to temporarily bring us to the next level. Living your life with this philosophy will help you respond better to what you viewed in the past as a failure. The next time something doesn't work out just say, "All right! That means I am now one step further ahead after learning "this".

Repeat this: ''I succeed at learning whatever I need to learn for my goal. I succeed at growing. I succeed at getting better and improving myself. Then I have another goal: To do it again differently and learn more."

OUR LANGUAGE LEADS
TO SELF-SABOTAGE

Why is it that, for some, specific behaviours, like snacking on junk food, eating a second helping when you are not hungry or indulging in sweets, are stronger than you? Do you believe chocolate has power over you? It is just a question of programming. People keep programming themselves to be weak with some particular behaviours. They say: "Oh for me, chips are my downfall", or "pie is my downfall." They are programming the brain that when they are in the bakery aisle at the grocery store, they will be weak and bring home a pie and eat it.

Doing tasks that draw you closer to clean living should be exciting. It doesn't have to be boring. There are some things you will love doing. Things that you don't need any "willpower" to accomplish. You will learn to program your brain to start loving and being good at what serves your health.

Question:

When you overeat or self-sabotage your health, who gives the call? Who is asking you to do so?

Answer:

Your brain.

What if your brain were conditioned to be healthy instead? Would it still give you the order to unleash these limiting behaviours? Why are you working against yourself?

You are self-sabotaging because you are focusing on the wrong thing: Not eating dessert, not ordering fries, not indulging on cheese, not watching television, not feeling heavy and overweight. Your brain hears **dessert, fries, cheese, television, heavy** and **overweight** and heads straight for these temptations every time. Your focus is on what to avoid rather than on what you can eat. You are going 'away from' something, instead of going towards something. Remember the 'kitchen NOT blue?'. Ask yourself the question: "What do you want instead?" Feed your personal assistant with the right orders.

You can see how our language is key to brain reprogramming.

LIMITING BELIEFS LEAD TO SELF-SABOTAGE

The combination of language and your experiences create limiting beliefs. You start creating these "truths" about clean living like: "eating healthy is a fad and doesn't taste good", "eating clean is expensive", "it takes too long to prepare the food", "I can never find the ingredients", the food is weird (like quinoa)", etc. We will help you break down these limiting beliefs later in this book.

You want to re-write your life. Create a new life, slowly, by creating new healthy habits, rather than going on yet another "miracle diet." How will you do it differently this time? You have been presented with the fundamental pieces you need in order to understand the system we are about to introduce you. Turn the page and enter Nathalie's THINK Yourself® D.N.A . System.

KEY CONCEPTS:

Positive Core Values and Good Intentions can be at the root of your self-sabotaging behaviour.

Identifying those values and intentions can help to turn the 'cause' into the 'cure'.

Past Experiences can cause self-sabotage. You become conditioned through your life experiences to expect and accept that life will go a certain way and you make your choices accordingly.

Your Limiting Beliefs can lead to self-sabotage. Your perception of yourself and the world around you governs much of how you interact with people and situations.

Your language can lead to self-sabotage. You become stuck in a bad feedback loop where habits and self-sabotage feed into each other. Creating healthier choices with your language can disrupt the feedback loop.

The way you think about success and your beliefs around your skills are causing you to self-sabotage your efforts to reach your career goals. YOU give the call.

CHAPTER 14:

THE NEUROLOGICAL LEVELS

"What lies behind you and what lies in front of you,
pales in comparison to what lies inside of you."

- Ralph Waldo Emerson

After an overview of the common obstacles you face when aiming for clean living, and how your brain works, we are now ready to introduce you to the foundational pieces of the D.N.A. System.

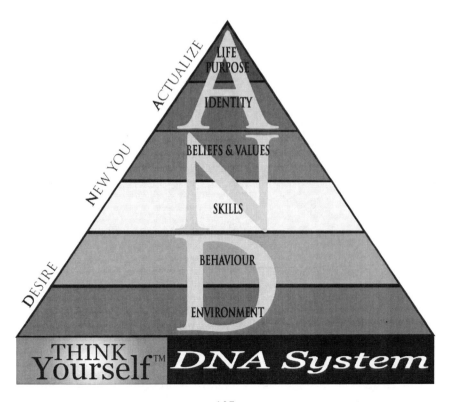

We will be explaining each of the levels through the lens of Robert Dilt's Neurological Levels. Robert Dilt's pyramid of Neurological Levels is an effective tool to help you better see who you are on the inside, which is often reflected in how you show up on the outside. The last decade of neuroscience research has discovered that your brain, previously thought to be rigid and unchanging, is actually malleable and capable of change (think neuroplasticity).

What does that mean for you? It means that, with greater awareness and understanding of how you are 'wired', coupled with consistent and repeated effort, you can 'change your stars' and 'change your fate!' You are not just the sum of your parts. You can choose to reorganize your bits and pieces and reinvent a much larger and more successful version of yourself.

LEVEL ONE: ENVIRONMENT

Your Environment is where you live, play, work and also includes your greater surroundings. It is a combination of the places you go and the people with whom you interact. In the material world, people often try to identify themselves by the type of car they drive, the neighbourhood in which they live or the type of office they have. None of these represent who you really are. These are just elements of your environment. Becoming identified with your environment can be positive if the environment supports you in a healthy way. Sometimes you can become over-identified with your environment, or place the wrong importance on the environment, which does not support you in a healthy way.

As an example of looking into environment to fix a client's problem, you can refer to the example of Tosca's client where the whole family was overweight because of their environment: What was in their fridge and their kitchen was part of an unhealthy environment for this family. The parents were obese, and they would continually order take out. When Tosca first went to their house, there was a stack of pizza boxes up to her shoulder. The refrigerator was loaded with pop and it was absent of vegetables. Tosca taught the family how to surround themselves with clean food including soups, turkey meat loaf, clean, homemade pasta sauces, a water cooler, and vegetables. In his worst days, the husband had to wear sleep apnea headgear to bed, because he weighed over 300 lbs and had a hard time breathing at night. This even affected his desire to make love to his wife because he felt he did not have enough oxygen capacity to perform the task. He lost half of that weight to now weigh a healthy 150 lbs and competed in his first triathlon, all in one year. His marriage is stronger than ever. The wife competed in an Ironman and the children no longer have behavioural problems at school. The clean environment that resulted from Tosca's guidance positively affected everyone in the family. The children lost excess weight, slept better and did better at school.

The family's health problems were directly related to their environment. Everyone from mom to dad to children, was always in a hurry. "OMG I am hungry, let's pick up the phone and order takeout!" The family did not prioritize the value of food.

If your environment supports you, you can start to embrace your own unique strengths. You can unravel and disengage from impairments to your growth and success. Sometimes you realize you have placed the wrong people, places and situations in your environment, or maybe once they were very right, but no longer serve your new positive initiatives.

Successful people surround themselves with an environment that supports their strong vision. Your success starts to become inevitable when you intentionally choose the right people, places and things, and build your new vision from the ground up.

LEVEL TWO:
BEHAVIOUR

Your behaviour is how you interact with family, friends and everyone else in life. It is what an observer may see, hear or feel when watching you engaged in a particular activity. Sometimes your behaviour can vary, depending on your circumstances. When you feel confident and comfortable, your behaviour will reflect that. If you feel unsure, threatened or nervous, your behaviour reflects that as well.

Sometimes your behaviour is consistent with the success you say you want, and other times it is not. When it is not, it is often because change needs to happen at a different level. Implementing a 'clean living strategy' won't be effective if the problem lies at the level of 'Beliefs and Values' or 'Identity'

If the problem is rooted in the values or beliefs layer it cannot be fixed at the behavioural level. If a problem resides in the identity or the belief system of a person, that is where the problem needs to be addressed. This explains why some of your past attempts at clean living have failed. It is because those behaviours were not addressed at the appropriate level. If you believe you are overweight because of genetics —beliefs and values level — then eating well and exercising - both behaviours—will not fix the problem. You will keep self-sabotaging yourself until you correct the beliefs.

Sometimes it is about disengaging from an old habit or way of being in the world, and consciously choosing to adopt new choices that are in alignment with your projected goal.

When your mind and habits are out of alignment with your dreams of living healthy, they don't fit and are not sustainable. If you behaviour is out of alignment with your dreams of clean living, you cannot create a strong present and future reality. Tosca worked with a woman who was constantly reaching for soda. She was feeling jittery, had restless leg syndrome, was losing her hair and had "menopot" which is the collection of fat around the middle. She was drinking "diet" soda thinking it was good for her because it was "diet". Over the course of a very busy work day at her law office, she would consume as many as five or six "diet" sodas every day. She did not realize she was doing anything wrong until Tosca made her do a food journal and track everything she ate as well as her hydration. Once she saw the black and white of it, it was easy to switch her to water can clean out her body. She just didn't know. The problem was at the behaviour level and by fixing the behaviour, she fixed the problem.

LEVEL THREE: CAPABILITIES AND SKILLS

Capability is the sum total of your skills, what you're good at and whether or not you have innate capabilities and/or learned skills for dealing appropriately with issues. Your skill set develops as you age and as a result of your life experiences. When you use your skills and do what you are good at, you feel in greater harmony with yourself. When using your skills, you avoid that sense of wasting your talent. When you are not good at something, you often give up and quickly use the "oh, well, that's not for me". It is similar to when an infant is learning to walk and continually falls. That child falls many times before being successful. It takes hundreds of attempts and weeks before a child can learn how to make it happen. Remember, no child has ever said: "Oh, well, I will just crawl for the rest of my life." The stakes are high and there is no quitting when it comes to that particular life skill. It is an essential one. So is being healthy. You must treat your learning about clean living in the same way an infant treats learning how to walk. Keep doing it over and over. With every effort, it becomes more deeply ingrained in our brains until it ultimately becomes a lifestyle.

This relates to the act of acquiring and preparing food. You may find the thought of looking for a meal, the ingredients and even the preparation of food, to be highly stressful activities. It explains a phenomenon that is happening today. People are spending more time at restaurants, buying frozen prepared food, ordering take-out, and eating at what has newly been coined a "grocerant", where they sit and eat prepared food at the grocery store. The process of getting food and preparing it has become overly stressful. Often, we default to: "Because I don't know, I don't do."

Cooking used to be taught at school in Home Economics classes. It used to be that you learned how to eat and cook at the elbow of your parents. You would likely have been involved in the process. This is changing. Since your parents eat out more frequently, as statistics show, they themselves often don't know how to cook. The model children follow today is what is demonstrated at home: how to buy already prepared food or how to pick up the phone and order home delivery.

To be sure, early efforts at cooking, just like when you learned how to walk, may end in a somewhat edible meal or complete failure. That is to be expected. If you persevere and teach yourself the necessary skills, you will improve. There is a strong tendency instead to abort mission, and retreat to the comfort zone. Improving your kitchen skills, including meal planning, food shopping and food preparation is easy and learnable. It is just a skill. Just like when you changed your flip phone to a smart phone. Treat your goal the same way. Trust that you will learn it and become good at it.

In Tosca's household, her mission was to teach her four daughters how to confidently cook, seven main dishes by the time they left the house to go to University. It is a life skill she felt was critical to their emancipation. Tosca's children grew up watching her cook. Her kitchen is always a happy place, not only during celebrations and regular meal times, but especially when life becomes stressful. Her daughters know how to nourish themselves well using clean living principles, because they had basic training in the kitchen at Tosca's elbow. They have confidence in their culinary skills and experience the joy associated with owning a "skill".

Your skills give you confidence and strength. We will teach you clean living skills you can perfect in order to fully immerse yourself into clean living. You don't have to have grown up in Tosca's household in order to master these skills. When you feel capable and skillful, you also feel knowledgeable. This leads to a greater state of empowerment. At this level, you experience greater confidence and proficiency which lead to success.

When you 'live' more authentically in the first two levels (of the D.N.S. system), it is reflected in the life choices you make. By releasing toxic environments and behaviours that no longer serve you, and replacing them with those that do, you experience a release of vital energy to pursue your goals and dreams with more clarity and a renewed sense of possibility. When you actively choose what you allow into your environment and the behaviours you wish to embrace you become more skillful, and in so doing, you send a strong signal that you feel ready and capable of doing more.

Remember the family who had an environment problem as a result of a fridge loaded with sodas and kitchen cluttered with pizza boxes? When Tosca replaced the sodas with the water cooler, it applied an environmental solution to an environmental problem. They also had a skill problem. No-one knew how to cook. They only knew how to order pizza. When Tosca came into the household and showed them how to make some of her simple Eat Clean® recipes, like easy spaghetti sauce, the family began to learn how to cook and heal themselves. It is the learning of these clean living life skills that set the family and you up for success.

LEVEL FOUR:
BELIEFS AND VALUES

Whether you believe something is possible or impossible, whether you believe it is necessary or unnecessary, whether or not you feel motivated about something is driven by what is imprinted in your unconscious. Level Four Beliefs and Values highlights the significance of this. What you believe is true, in your own representational systems, and shapes you. Beliefs are at the base of your habits (good or bad). They are the main focus in the NEW YOU section of the System. You need to change your old negative beliefs in order to replace them with beliefs that will serve you better.

You will know you have stepped into the sticky realm of Beliefs and Values if you find yourself saying: "I just keep doing THAT THING I said I wasn't going to do." Your choices defy logic as your unconscious mind rules, and the unconscious mind is often governed by negative emotion.

We have given you some examples where clients had environmental, behavioural, or skill problems. These three are not the most common. Most people's problems reside in their beliefs, values and identity levels. The closer to the base of the pyramid, the easier the problem is to fix. When you run out of milk, the solution is to go out and buy some. The closer the problem is to the identity level (at the top), the more you see it as a real problem. An easy example of this is when someone has a self-confidence problem (belief) and to give themselves prestige and power, they buy themselves an expensive sports car. The problem lies in the belief level (self-confidence) but they are trying to fix it in the environment level (sports car). This does not work. Again, the problem needs to be addressed in the area from which it originates.

Your beliefs and values are guiding every one of your actions. When your beliefs make you grow and give you a fulfilling life, you can thank them for making life easy for you. When, on the other hand, your beliefs make you see the world from a negative angle, you wish you could change them. The beliefs that are not serving you are called *limiting beliefs*.

Here are some examples:

BEING HEALTHY IS HARD.

Says who? Try being ill for a while and tell us which one is worse? What if you choose to believe it is easy to be healthy? If you believe that being healthy is hard, then you are telling your brain this same thing and programming it to make being healthy difficult for you. Every time you think about this statement, or every time you say it out loud, you are providing a reason for your brain to make it hard for you.

EATING CLEAN IS EXPENSIVE

This belief is not serving you. The idea behind mind shifting is not to make you live on a tight budget or to teach you how to be wise with your food budget. Instead it will teach you that you always have everything you need and that you can Eat Clean® on any budget.

IN MY FAMILY, WE WERE TOLD THAT A GOOD MEAL NEEDED TO INCLUDE MEAT, STARCHES, SAUCES AND DESSERT.

The science of this book is based on modeling. You can choose to model your parents or you can choose to model your healthy friends or anyone who knows how to prepare delicious clean foods.

THAT IS HOW I AM; I AM DOOMED TO STAY THIS WAY.

You have your own character and excel at your skills. What are your dreams? What if you want to be more of this or less of that? You can visualize yourself being your best. Any skill can be learned and any behaviour can be adopted.

NO DIET WORKS FOR ME. NO MATTER WHAT I DO, I CAN'T LOSE WEIGHT.

Nothing ever worked? Ever? What would happen if it did? Have you considered that this belief, and its constant repetition in your head, might be the main reason that has prevented you from achieving your ideal weight and wellness all these years?

I DON'T HAVE WILLPOWER SO I CAN'T STOP EATING SUGAR, SALTY, CRUNCHY, WINE AND CHOCOLATE.

How does not having willpower cause you to choose to believe that you can't succeed? Are these things connected? Could willpower be an invention that we use as an excuse for our incorrect programming? The very thing you feel that you can't live without is likely the very thing that is preventing you from achieving whatever wellness or physical goals you desire for yourself. When do you decide that it is time for your fix? What if we could re-wire your brain to have a different *want* at this exact moment?

EATING CLEAN® IS A LOT OF WORK.

And being overweight and unwell is not a lot of work? How about the hours you spent trying to fix problems that occurred because you are not healthy? Many people who do not eat clean opt out of life, passing on a hike, not putting on a bathing suit and enjoying the beach because of their unhealthy lifestyle. They won't even go to a party because they can't find a dress or a suit that fits.

I HAVE CHILDREN, SO I CANNOT EAT CLEAN®.

Your children are the most powerful reason to eat clean. Their future wellness depends on you. Everything you teach them at the childhood level, they will take into adulthood. Teach them how to Eat Clean® and live clean to set them up for success for the rest of their lives. Isn't that our job as parents?

Whether you think you can or think you can't,
you are absolutely right.

- Henry Ford

LEVEL FIVE: IDENTITY

Identity is who you are. It is your self-esteem, your sense of self and what you identify with. This can include identifying with your job, marriage, religion, etc. It can also include how you interpret events in terms of your self-worth and what you think you deserve or not.

You may be familiar with the expression, 'I AM a morning person.' This is a deep set belief about who you are at your core. You are not born to be morning or evening people. You choose to be more effective in the morning (or not) because you think it is so, act so and articulate this 'fact' to others. Saying the words: 'I AM' a morning person is a symbol of a deeply ingrained belief. It is much different from saying, "I work well in the morning" or "I get up early" which are behavioural affirmations and not identity-related.

Understanding each level of yourself and identifying where the problems exist within you is a potent step towards fixing them. When you hear people say, "I am healthy," it's important to know that the words "I AM" are infinitely powerful. Saying "I am" means they don't only think of themselves as living healthy (behaviour), they say I AM, which refers to their deeply ingrained beliefs at the level of their identity, that they are already healthy.

When you implement change, the higher you go on the neurological pyramid, the deeper you need to dig into your ingrained beliefs about yourself in order to make change. By changing cars or clothes, you are only changing an environmental aspect of your life. But by changing who you are, you lose, in some aspect, a portion of yourself.

Most people are wary of change, as no one wants to lose their sense of self. Who are you going to be if you cannot be who you thought you were all your life? That is when re-writing your software and deciding what and who you want to be is an empowering tool that allows you to let go of your old self and embrace your new identity.

Whenever you say: "I Am" you are referring to the Identity level, down in your deepest structure. However, before you got to your deepest self, your identity, you started at a lower level of consciousness. To be fulfilled at this level, you need to be able to be your true self.

Doctor Wayne Dyer created a mediation system using the powerful "I Am" words. I am "that" I am...[6]

This Moses Code Meditation is a powerful tool to rewire your brain with positive thinking through repeating the "I am that I am" mantra, while listening to this beautiful meditation. When you say the mantra, you insert a word you wish to be, like "powerful" or "healthy" in place of the word that. It would sound like this:

"I am powerful, I am."

"I am beautiful, I am."

"I am healthy, I am."

---

6   www.drwaynedyer.com/mosescodemeditation

LEVEL SIX:
LIFE PURPOSE

When all the layers of the pyramid are aligned, when you live in a supportive environment, doing what you are good at and following your beliefs and values, you feel like you are being your true self and living your real-life purpose. Your life purpose is the reason you were put on this earth. What is beyond yourself? Who else are you serving with your life? What cause is close to your heart?

You can use the D.N.A. model to recognize how the various levels interact and how they are related. It provides a means of recognizing at which level a problem is occurring and recognizing the most appropriate level at which to target the solution.

Here is one last example:

Tosca has worked with a client for a number of years. She is a big fan of Eating Clean®, shops for the right kind of food, exercises, follows clean living principles. Everything on the outside looks perfect. Yet, there is an underlying current that prevents her from reaching her ideal weight despite her clean efforts. It turns out she wasn't living her life. She was living her husband's life. She had turned herself off and become the "model" wife her husband was looking for, doing what he wanted her to do. She became introverted, unhappy and absent from reality. She was not doing anything for herself. Tosca taught her how to find meaning in activities outside of her relationship that gave her joy. When she tapped into long quiet elements of herself and began to express and act on them, she felt more complete in herself.

There is no reason to compete with others (only ourselves). You can celebrate your unique gifts as well as those of others. You can also recognize that there is a unifying oneness between us all. In Life Purpose, you understand that you are co-creators and co-conspirators in Life. You know why you are here, what you are here to do, whom you are here to serve, and you live your Life's Purpose. This adds up to living in alignment with your true self.

People are naturally drawn to you when you live this way because you are living your Why with a strong sense of conviction. That inspires confidence, trust and safety. People want to be around you because your wellness emanates from a deep place within yourself. You are unwavering and uncompromising in your purpose and commitment to living from a place of authenticity.

KEY CONCEPTS:

THE FOUNDATION OF THE THINK Yourself® D.N.A. SYSTEM

Your brain classifies information into different levels in the brain.

Environment. Behaviours. Skill. Beliefs and Values. Identity. Life Purpose.

You need to identify where the problems are and fix them where they originate.

Beliefs and Values along with Identity are the main areas where the deeper problems reside.

Going through each layer will reprogram your brain to get you transformational results.

.

PART 5

THE "D"

CHAPTER 15:

DESIRE

*"The first principle of success is desire -
knowing what you want. Desire is the planting
of your seed."*

- Robert Collier

The first part of the D.N.A. System is DESIRE. This section revolves around the first two neurological levels: Environment and Behaviour.

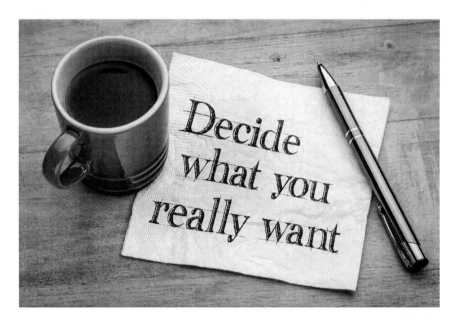

Remember in chapter one we gave you the analogy of the kitchen renovation? The DESIRE part of the system is the first step towards getting your full "kitchen" installed. Assume that you have an open budget. No restrictions. Give yourself lots of choices. Make it amazing and compelling!

This technique of writing down your goal(s) is not something new. You have probably already made a 'list' or 'vision board'. These are fine tools but useless if they are not followed. These vision boards and smart goals are just like the folder you will make before starting your "kitchen" renovation. However, you cannot cook in a folder, nor can you entertain people in a folder. A folder is not a kitchen, just like your vision board is not a clean living lifestyle.

Our system is based on how your brain processes information. It follows the layers of your internal reality. The D.N.A. System offers you two more actionable steps. This book continues where most other literature ends. Deciding what you want is only the first step. A folder full of images and thoughts is just that. A folder. Your folder full of images and thoughts needs to be implemented in order to take life. Let's start at the beginning and let's start filling up that folder.

As you do so you will become aware of your current situation, what surrounds you and what physical evidence you will want to experience when you reach your goal. You will start replacing your old behaviours with what serves you better. You will define what clean living is for you. You will be asked a multitude of questions with the intention of generating ideas that will allow you to elicit your perfect outcome and write your daily affirmation. This will serve as a reference, a plan, a map, and a vision of your positive outcome.

Finally, this section will invite you to generate exactly what you want, and to aim for a multitude of choices and opportunities to follow the real intent behind your desires. Enjoy the process of discovering yourself and what you truly want.

KEY CONCEPTS:

DESIRE DEFINE

The first part of the D.N.A System is DESIRE. This section of the book will help you define what you want.

CHAPTER 16:

WHAT DO YOU WANT?

"You can become whoever you want to be. You can do what you want to do."

- Jake Paul

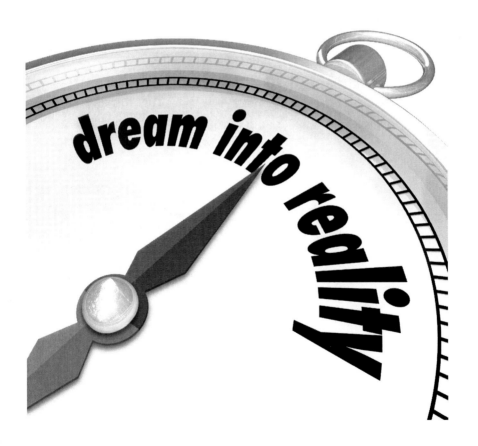

The next few chapters will help you create a compelling image of yourself achieving your goal(s). We will offer you a series of questions. These are the start of how you will reprogram your brain to achieve what you want. As you work through the questions, pay attention to three factors that need to happen for the process to work. These factors are the physical responses that need to happen in your brain. You need to *see it*, to *hear it* and to *feel it*. Each of you is biologically unique therefore, you will also have a preferred sense that you rely on for information processing, but you must take of senses into consideration.

VISUAL

You will visualize yourself having achieved your goal(s). We invite you to time-shift yourself in the future to a moment where your goal(s) have been accomplished. The questions will generate images in your mind which we recommend you embrace and allow. The value of these images lies in their details. The more detailed you are, the more likely you will be successful in reprograming your brain. Allow yourself to immerse yourself in the visualization process.

AUDITORY

Hearing the answers in your head will start to re-program your self-talk. The voice you hear talking to yourself on a regular basis can be managed so it can change the conversation you are having with yourself. Saying out loud what you want will also have a positive reinforcing effect. Imagining what other people will be telling you once you have achieved your goal(s) will also contribute to your success.

Be careful what you say! Your mind is always
listening. - Unknown

KINESTHETIC

Your brain also needs to feel how it will feel when you have achieved your goal(s) in order to prime it for success. Generating the feelings of success and immersing yourself in the outcome will play a significant role in your brain programming. There is value in writing down what arises for you during the process. You learn by putting things on paper or by typing it. Writing enhances the success experience. Science reveals that you are fifty percent more likely to be successful in any ventures, including brain programming, when you commit your goals to paper (ref. www.goalband.co.uk). The reasons for this are many. Writing down your dreams, goals and ideas helps you brainstorm more deeply into what these can look like. You will also learn more because areas of the brain associated with learning work better when writing is involved. You will also remember more and won't be easily distracted. Writing cleans up your brain because writing takes words, thoughts and ideas out of your brain and gives them a place to live other than your gray matter. You will be beautifully set up for success.

You can download the free THINK Yourself® CLEAN workbook on www.thinkyourself.com where we suggest you write down your answers to get the full value.

The temptation may be to keep on reading the questions without stopping to process and answer. We encourage you to pause after each question, see what you need to see, hear what you need to hear and feel what you need to feel. Then move on to the next question.

There is a marked difference between READING and DOING. Take the time to really DO the processes and answer the questions suggested... just reading them is not enough. You want to take the time you need and get the full benefit of generating the answers for each question.

There will be different types of activities suggested throughout the system. You will have your favourite ones. You may need to close your eyes and see what that looks like for you. You may choose to write. You may want to sit back and think about it. You may want to read them out loud. Answer the questions when you are relaxed and have time to do them with purpose.

Tosca had a client who wanted to get healthy. She did not really know what aspects needed to be cleaned up. She just knew she was not happy where she was. She felt terrible and had a poor relationship with her mother. Tosca explained that clean living is a lifestyle based on eating clean, exercise and emotional self-care. At the beginning of the process, all the client could manage (imagine, hear, see, feel) was to get healthy. With Tosca's help she removed damaging foods from her client's diet and helped her clean up her kitchen and environment. The client noticed how good she felt and how much more energy she had. She was ready to add the exercise part into the mix. She began by walking longer and longer distances that eventually led to running and finally to marathons. Then it led to emotional self-care. In the emotional self-care process Tosca established, she taught her client how to meditate and then to sit with her thoughts immediately after meditating so that she could spend some time journaling. Tosca's client is now healthy in every way including being reunited with her estranged mother. Life for her feels good again.

At the beginning of the process, you may not have the full picture with all the details of what you want your clean life to look like. Start with one thing at a time. Once you get to the next level, go back to the questions and create another goal for yourself. And repeat.

KEY CONCEPTS:

Three factors (visual, auditory and kinesthetic) will influence positively your ability to create your dream.

When you create your desire, make sure to include details about what it will look like, what you will hear and what how you will feel. Creating your dreams in three dimensions will create a compelling image for your brain to already feel the end-result.

CHAPTER 17:

STAY AWAY FROM WHAT YOU DON'T WANT

"Nobody can motivate himself in a positive direction by continually using negative words."

- John C Maxwell

When you ask people what they want or desire, most respond with a negative affirmation stating what they don't want. They want to stop being sick. They want to stop feeling stressed. They don't want to be overweight. They don't want to be stressed. They want to stop being impatient with their kids. They are tired of rushing everywhere all the time. They speak in negatives. The real question is: "What do you want?"

Defining your desire is crucial. It is as if you were to ask your interior designer, who is helping you remodel your kitchen, that you want them to paint the kitchen 'not blue'.

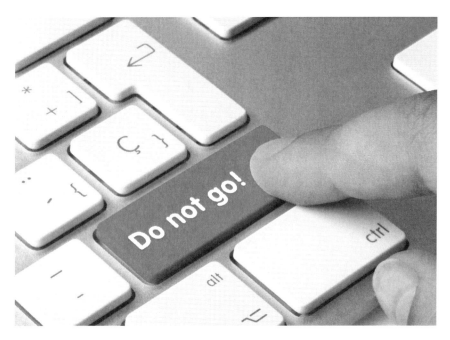

If you use negative words to say what you want, you obtain exactly that result. For example: You glance at your lunch in the fridge when you grab the milk for your coffee in the morning and you tell yourself: "I can't forget my lunch tomorrow. If I do, I will have to eat out again." You just programmed your brain to 'forget my lunch' and 'eat out'. The day after, you show up at the office and you forgot your lunch that you had actually 'programmed yourself to forget'.

The words you use to make your demands to your brain matter. Whatever you focus on, you will get.

You have learned that your personal assistant is always listening. Your brain is making you right. If somewhere in your mind you have a belief that you're a loser, and your brain hears it over and over, then your brain will make you right. If for the past 15 years you have been looking at yourself in the mirror every day telling yourself: "I am overweight!" or "I am so tired" or "I am a failure", these discriminating thoughts, the brain hears them loudly and clearly, and it does everything it can to make you right!!! If you focus on not being a failure and not being tired and overweight, your brain hears *failure, tired* and *overweight*.

With a mindset of being a failure (your words), and your brain wanting to make you right and make sure that you are a failure because you asked for it, it will never ask you to do anything that could make your life bloom; your brain is doing everything it can to make you right and keep you struggling, because that is what you are conditioned to be. You are thinking about yourself as a person having no willpower when it comes to food and that is the way it is.

Imagine that you do very well with your clean living efforts for a while. You start preparing meals in advance and take a healthy lunch to work. You eat healthy snacks, and you start having more energy, being more focused and losing weight. Then your brain begins to panic. It says: "oh no!... What is going on?... She is getting healthy and focused and she is supposed to be tired and failing (because your messages to yourself said that). What can I do...to make her right about being a failure? Oh... here is a chocolate bar, I'm going to make her eat that." You feel you are sabotaging yourself, but in fact, you are just following the exact instructions you gave yourself.

Here is an example that has probably already happened to you, millions of times. You opened the fridge, looking for the water jug, and did not see it at first glance. You said out loud: "I am so blind, what's wrong with me?" and you kept repeating it in your brain: "I am so blind, it is probably empty in the sink, or in the dishwasher." Then your spouse comes behind you and takes it out of the fridge, right in front of your eyes. It was on the shelf, at eye-level right in front of you but you had stopped your brain from seeing it. When you started saying 'I am blind', you were making yourself right by not seeing it. The brain always listens!

Your brain will always make you right. You must be careful with the thoughts and words you put into your brain. You have to be careful about what you want to be right about.

Do many of your thoughts tend to use the phrase 'do-not'? You try to stay away from what you don't want instead of thinking with positive words. Focus on the right things with the proper mindset and your brain will make it easy for you to accomplish anything.

In the next chapter, we will ask you what you want. Make sure you remember to respond in the positive.

KEY CONCEPTS:

When asked what you want, you usually respond with what you don't want.

Using do-not in your language is not serving your cause even if your intentions are positive.

When programming yourself with what you don't want, your brain is creating a model of reality that is not serving you and is making you right about it.

CHAPTER 18:

ENVIRONMENT
WHERE ARE YOU NOW?

*"You are the average of the five people you
spend the most time with."*

- Jim Rohn

Let's start your work at the bottom of the pyramid, in the Environment level of the brain. The first step is to define your current situation and your surroundings.

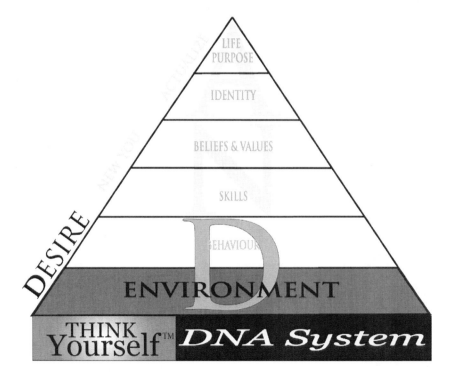

We will help you discover where you are 'now' and guide you towards where you want to be. At the base of the System, you start by answering questions about your environment. Environment is the base that influences the rest of the layers of your brain. The work ahead will prepare you to choose the appropriate foundation for your life. What or whom you allow into your life gives you clues as to how you feel about yourself, both positively and negatively. This awareness is crucial and foundational to clean living on every level.

If you constantly hang around with people who are lowering your "average" you will eventually become them. Even if you are the one that orders a salad at the pub while everyone else is having burgers and fries, it won't be long before you are tempted to join them. By being around others who do not value clean living, you lower the bar of wellness for yourself. You only try as hard as you have to. You feel that with the pasta, you are still making healthier choices than your friends are. The comparison to others can play tricks on you.

KEY CONCEPTS:

ENVIRONMENT

There are clues in your environment that guide you to understanding what you want.

This is the starting point and foundation for all future work in this book.

CHAPTER 19:

MYTHS
FAT

*"The great enemy of the truth is very often not
the lie, deliberate, contrived and dishonest, but
the myth, persistent, persuasive and unrealistic."*

- John F. Kennedy

Your environment contains abundant information about food that can add to your confusion. This chapter will review myths and trends related to fat.

FAT STARVATION

Fat starvation is an outcome resulting from the myth that fat makes us fat. Going back to our ancestors, who ate 40% to 80% fat in their diet, and experienced optimal health with no dental caries, no major diseases and no fertility issues, we can observe the powerful nutritional value of fat. It should also be stated that there was no obesity in those ancestral cultures, since food was much more difficult to obtain, unlike the 24/7 presence of food in today's society. Blaming fat for your weight and health problems is a mistake.

Many today are starving themselves by not consuming enough healthy fats. This is fat starvation. Fat is the signal that triggers much of your eating biochemistry. Fat is needed to trigger the brain to either start or stop eating, otherwise dysfunctional eating results, as seen previously when the functions of ghrelin and leptin were explained. Highly dis-regulated eating functions including the extremes, of anorexia, bulimia and morbid obesity, are rampant in society today.

For the first time in history, there is less starvation thanks to the abundance of calories available, but those calories are devoid of nutrients, particularly when it comes to fat. We need fat to absorb certain nutrients in the body, specifically, vitamins A, D, E and K which are fat soluble. Protein also cannot be properly absorbed without fat. Fat creates all hormones in the body and is necessary for proper brain and nervous function. There is a resurgence of malnutrition and disease in modern society as a result of these empty calories.

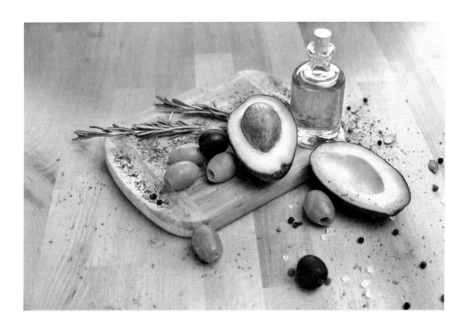

MYTH:
A LIGHT OLIVE OIL IS BETTER
THAN REGULAR OLIVE OIL.

An oil is an oil. It will always be 9 calories per gram of fat (and we will treat coconut oil separately). There is no oil that is light. Marketing companies are trying to trick your mind. When you see "light", you may think it is better for you. It isn't. You may cook with olive oil already, so it is important to know how oils are manufactured so that you don't harm yourself. In the same way you have switched your white, refined flour to whole grain flour, and table salt to sea salt, it is now time to switch your refined oil to an unrefined version.

There are different oil manufacturing processes. Ideally oil should be transformed as little as possible. Virgin, first-cold-pressed oils have been pressed at cold temperatures, slowly, to maintain the good properties and vitamins in the natural oil. This is the best oil to consume as part of a clean living lifestyle.

Other oils are processed rapidly, creating heat in the high-speed process. Heat negatively affects the properties of oil. Manufacturers often add solvents to make the olive sweat more, helping to extract more oil from it. The olive is pressed repeatedly until there is nothing left. The solvent will then need to be removed.

The process used to remove the solvent is called the refining process. As the solvent is removed, nutrients including essential fatty acids (EFAs) and vitamins (if they are not already dead because of the heat applied) are also removed. Once refined, the resulting clear, drab oily substance is then given artificial color and taste (otherwise you would not believe that it is actually sunflower oil or canola oil). It is at this stage that the word "light" comes in. A little bit of flavor added becomes a light olive oil. It does not mean it's lower in fat. It means it tastes less like olive oil.

Any oil that has been refined or hydrogenated to any degree is not healthy for you. These oils include canola oil, grapeseed oil, safflower oil and soy oil. Even an organic version of any of these will not be healthy if it is refined.

MYTH:
AN EXTRA-VIRGIN OIL IS
BETTER THAN A VIRGIN OIL

Virgin olive oil is an oil that has not been refined, and still has all its healthful properties. What about extra virgin? Is it more virgin than just a virgin oil? No. The word "extra" refers to many taste characteristics that describe the quality of the fruit that is pressed (mainly olive). One of these elements is the amount of acidity in the olive. If the acidity is below 0.8, then an olive can be considered extra virgin olive oil. But it only refers to olives.

Some marketing companies have started to put the word 'extra' on many different types of oils (such as canola, sunflower, and coconut). Those manufacturers are trying to trick you. The strategy is that the words 'extra virgin' imply something better to you. If it is better, they think you will buy their oil. Now you know! Don't be fooled again. The words 'extra' and 'virgin' are two different things. A virgin oil means that the oil is unrefined, first-cold-pressed or cold-extraction. These are all synonyms. That adjective can be applied for canola, sunflower, walnut, sesame, hazelnut or any oil. An extra virgin oil is firstly 'virgin', see above, and also 'extra' which refers to olive oil only, and it's mainly a measure of acidity and taste.

ESSENTIAL FATTY ACIDS (EFA'S).

Omega 3, 6 and 9 essential fatty acids are necessary for optimal wellness. They are called essential fatty acids because the body needs them and can't manufacture them on its own. Essential fatty acids must come from your diet. You need to make sure that the oil you are about to buy and consume still has the essential fatty acids in it and that the EFA's are still alive and will give you the benefits you need. In order to recognize an oil that is more likely to have healthy living EFA's in it, you must know that they are fragile. Oils are easily and quickly affected by air, time, and heat.

HEAT

Look for the words virgin, first-cold-pressed, cold-extraction. Because oils are affected by heat, you must ensure that the oil was extracted without heat. If you see for example a mention of mechanically pressed or expeller-pressed, it doesn't tell you that it was extracted without heat. All it tells you is that a machine extracted it. Avoid these.

AIR

Look for a dark glass bottle that protects the oil. What would be the point of extracting an oil at very low temperature and then putting it in a plastic see-through bottle that could compromise the integrity of the EFA's? You can eliminate many players right in the oil aisle at the grocery store just by looking at the bottles and where they are positioned on the shelf. If it's a clear plastic bottle, sitting near lights, consider this a red flag. Don't buy these oils.

TIME

EFA's are alive because they have been preserved in the manufacturing process. The product you buy also needs to have an expiration date because the oil has living components in it. You want to know how long these elements will be alive. Would you buy milk if it had no expiration date on it? If you buy an oil with no expiration date, chances are it is already dead or rancid —and contains no good properties for you.

COCONUT OIL

Coconut oil has the natural property of turning to a liquid state at more than 25 degrees, which means that it becomes liquid very fast. There is no need to heat it in order to melt it. Just a stir will do the trick. That property is exactly what made it so popular about 15-20 years ago when researchers realized that coconut oil was a saturated fat (solid fat) that became liquid inside your body (which is approximately 27 degrees) and did not clog the arteries unlike margarine, butter, shortening, lard, and solid fat in meat.

Use coconut oil as you would a solid fat to make piecrust, in your baking, to butter your toast, grilled cheese sandwiches and more. Coconut oil doesn't clog your arteries since it becomes a liquid immediately in your body and is readily absorbed thus. Since coconut oil is a saturated fat and not as fragile as the polyunsaturated and monounsaturated fats, it has a high smoke point. The high smoke point is ideal for cooking because it assures that no free radicals or "trans fats" are created. Both free radicals and trans fats are initiators of disease.

When you eat you need to transform your food into energy in order to be able to absorb it. Coconut oil is a medium chain triglyceride, which means, it is energy already transformed into readily accessible energy for your body's use. Coconut oil is the preferred fuel for the heart. Your body gets immediate energy from it as soon as you eat it, which makes your metabolism run faster. When your metabolism runs faster, you then burn more calories, which can be associated with weight loss. Coconut oil has become very popular as an energy booster for athletes and *the* "diet" tool for people wanting to lose weight. Coconut oil also has less calories than other oils with only six calories per gram while all others contain 9.[7]

Coconut oil is the only oil to contain Laureic Acid. Only breast milk contains as much anti-viral, anti-microbial and anti-bacterial properties. Coconut oil will prevent you from becoming ill and if you do happen to fall ill, it will not necessarily repair the cell, but it will keep it from degenerating more. There is an abundance of scientific studies available supporting the health properties of coconut oil. It is interesting to note that in countries where coconut oil consumption is ubiquitous, there are far lower rates of heart disease, AIDS, cancer and Alzheimer disease. Researchers are studying the use of coconut oil in cancer patients and those suffering from Alzheimer disease. When coconut oil is used on these patients it appears there is some effect on cancer cells, stopping their growth and brain cells stop degenerating with the use of this marvelous oil. As mentioned in the first few pages of the book, we are not doctors nor researchers and we are not making any claims.

To recap: virgin coconut oil is a solid fat that doesn't clog the arteries, it is a rich source of energy and an anti-viral, anti-bacterial and anti-microbial fat that promotes overall wellness. A therapeutic dose of coconut oil is three tablespoons per day. Cook your egg in it in the morning, add it to your smoothie, apply to Paleo Loaf or even smooth it on your body. It is an excellent personal lubricant to enhance sexual pleasure. Nathalie uses it to wash herself in the

---

7   Mary Enig and Sally Fallon Know Your Fats.

shower, mixed with instant coffee and olive oil - as a body scrub. Tosca uses coconut oil mixed with essential oils and sea salt as a delightful body scrub.

GUTTER OIL

As reported by the Washington Post and many other media sources since, gutter oil is heavily used in the Chinese street food vending market. Labourers are hired to go into garbage dumpsters, trash bins, gutters and sewers, collecting liquid and solid waste that contains used oil and animal parts. The collected material is boiled and sold to the general public and food vendors as oil. Apart from the obvious, that it is a disgusting and unhealthy practice, it is also a calculated, unscrupulous effort to deceive the consumer. Gutter oils contain all manner of pathogens and carcinogens that will only make the consumer ill.

Practices such as these in the inherent trickery in oil production forces you, the consumer, to be extra vigilant when purchasing oil of any kind. In general terms, be impeccable with your fat choices. In all living species, fat is the safe storage place for toxins. If you are eating fat, you may be getting an unwelcome dose of agents that will contribute to disease.

AVOCADO

Avocado is the new healthy fat. It is a berry fruit containing a single large seed. Interestingly, 'avocado' is the Mayan word for testicles. Avocado is a super food ideal for those who are on low fat diets. Avocado flesh is highly nutritious containing 215 calories (in a medium fruit) but thanks to the healthy fat, fiber and nutrient content, this food will actually help you lose weight. It is high in vitamins A, E, D and particularly vitamin K, and the fact that avocado has a high fat content, ensures you will absorb these fat-soluble nutrients. You can use it sweet or savory. It is highly versatile in your clean living kitchen as an ingredient.

CHOLESTEROL

It is often stated that cholesterol is bad for health and that it must be avoided at all cost. It is one of the main elements measured by doctors when you get your annual checkup. You may have been told by your physician that you need to lower your cholesterol, so you automatically assume it is a bad thing …

WHAT IS CHOLESTEROL?

Cholesterol is a molecule (a sterol) found in all animal cell membranes that allows the cell membrane to maintain integrity and fluidity. Not only is it important for cells to be able to change shape, unlike plants that are rigid, it also allows your body to convert steroid hormones, bile acids and vitamin D into more complex compounds so that your body can fully absorb from them.

That is why animal products contain cholesterol and plant products don't. If you are unsure as to whether a product is high in cholesterol or not, the easy way is to think about it is its' source. Is it a grain? Is it a plant? Is it a vegetable? Is it animal based? Which wouldn't contain LDL cholesterol? Consider which of these would contain cholesterol.

WHAT ARE THE TYPES OF CHOLESTEROL?

There are three types of cholesterol and an additional lipid that interact with them. The three types are: HDL high-density lipoprotein, LDL low-density lipoprotein and VLDL very low-density lipoprotein. Triglycerides, another type of lipid, interacts with them. We will address the two main types of cholesterol: HDL (known as the good cholesterol) and LDL (referred to as the bad one). Here is Nathalie's trick to remember which one is which: HDL = H = Healthy. LDL = L = Lousy.

Here is a way to understand cholesterol's role in your body. You have a long highway of tubes, veins and arteries making up your circulatory system. You are faced with different stresses in your life that can damage this circulatory system: high blood pressure, high blood sugar, poor diet, cigarettes, exposure to fiberglass and more. Each of these can nick the smooth inner layer of your arteries creating little 'holes' or irregularities in that inner layer.

LDL

When travelling through your body, the LDL cholesterol (the lousy one) notices these holes or irregularities and it starts to fill these holes. It's like putty that you put on drywall when there is a hole that needs to be filled. The LDL putty is also trying to regulate the shape of the arteries when there are fat deposits (like the fat present in most processed foods, on the side of a steak, and in hydrogenated fat and shortening). If there is a little lump of fat sitting in your artery, the LDL adds more putty (cholesterol) trying to create an even surface again. But this results in making the arteries smaller, and ultimately clogs them. This concept is known as plaque formation. LDL is really doing the job it was meant to do so blaming the presence of cholesterol in your blood is a lot like blaming the fire man for showing up at a fire. He didn't start the fire, but he has to do his job to put it out. Cholesterol didn't start the problem in your arteries, but your poor diet caused nicks that had to be repaired. The more cholesterol gets deposited on the inside of your arteries the narrower they become, leaving less space for the transportation of nutrients, blood and oxygen.

HDL

The good cholesterol travels around in your highway of arteries and notices the patching attempts made by the LDL. It stops at the intersections where the site of an LDL operation has happened, and it cleans up the mess left by the cholesterol. It is like a spatula that you use on your putty job when dry-walling. The HDL comes along and finishes the job that LDL started. Ideally, you would need more HDL than LDL since you want as many chances for your arteries to be clean and wide open. You also want your highways to transport as many nutrients and as much healthy blood as possible. Ultimately you want a higher ratio of HDL vs. LDL.

HOW DO WE LOWER OUR LDL AND INCREASE OUR HDL?

Exercise and living a smoke-free life will definitively help in lowering your LDL cholesterol. Eating less saturated fat and increasing consumption of monounsaturated fats and polyunsaturated fats (the Essential Fatty acids (EFA'S) known also as omega 3, 6 and 9) will also increase your HDL level. These types of fats can be found in extra virgin olive oil, which is also loaded with anti-oxidants that will lower your LDL cholesterol, virgin flaxseed oil, virgin GMO-free canola oil and virgin walnut oil. Whole grains will help lower your LDL cholesterol as well.

KEY CONCEPTS:

Healthy Fats are necessary in order to absorbs nutrients in our body.

Olive oil: When buying oils, look for cold-pressed virgin or extra virgin oils.

Avocado is the new healthy fat.

Cholesterol includes HDL and LDL. HLD is the healthy cholesterol that helps your system deliver nutrients tour blood and get rid of undesirable LDL.

CHAPTER 20:

MYTHS
CARBOHYDRATES

*"The three most harmful addictions are heroin,
carbohydrates, and a monthly salary."*

— *Nassim Nicholas Taleb*

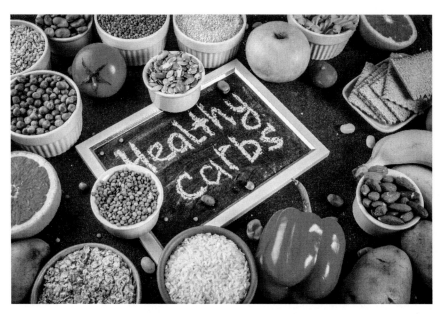

There has hardly been a food that has confused your thinking more than carbohydrates. Carbohydrates are a necessary macronutrient in the human diet if you hope to be optimally well in all areas. However, the mere mention of the word causes many to sweat, fearing the danger of weight gain. Where has the confusion come from?

Carbohydrates encompass a group of organic, mostly plant-based compounds found in food and living tissues. There are starches, sugars and cellulose in the carbohydrate group. Made of hydrogen, oxygen and water molecules, carbohydrates are broken down to create energy. They drive your human bus, if you will.

SIMPLE AND COMPLEX CLEAN CARBOHYDRATES

Think of carbohydrates as simple or complex. A simple carbohydrate breaks down very quickly while a complex carbohydrate will take longer to process. Tosca thinks of carbohydrates in this way: Simple carbohydrates are quick burning, much like paper when you start a fire. Sometimes you need the quick burning carbohydrates to fuel your efforts, like during a workout. You don't want to wait a long time to receive that energy. Complex carbohydrates take longer to burn, much like a log on a fire. Longer burning carbohydrates, like that big log on a fire, provide a longer, slower supply of energy. Complex carbohydrates take longer to break down because they usually have a fibrous element to them.

You need both types of carbohydrates to function optimally. In an emergency situation, simple carbohydrates fuel the rapid-fire actions and decision-making processes in the brain. Their value is in their quick breakdown so that you can access that fuel immediately. However, you also need slower burning carbs to fuel your activities over a longer period of time. This is useful when you are participating in endurance events or working hard in your garden or at work.

Optimal wellness and clean living require that you eat both simple and complex carbohydrates. The only carbohydrates you need to avoid are the 'dangerous' refined carbs. When you think about it, every carbohydrate started from a plant. The less it looks like its original plant-form, the more highly refined it is, the more dangerous it is for your health. Aim for carbs that are the least transformed as possible. In its whole form, coming directly from the plant, a carbohydrate does little harm. It delivers natural energy, vitamins, fiber, enzymes, minerals and other nutrients. Taken as a whole, carbohydrates provide us with much that bolsters an optimally well person.

REFINED CARBOHYDRATES

Carbohydrates are found in all plants, but they are also found in a cereal box, the cookie tin, ice cream, crackers, and numerous processed foods.

When plants are stripped down, the entity they once were, is destroyed resulting in the loss of nutritional value. The result is often a dangerous pseudo-food that robs the body of its constituent building blocks and ultimately your wellness.

In today's world all carbohydrates have been given a bad name. The confusion lies in the fact that the same name 'carbohydrate' is used to describe the goodness of an apple as well as that of a chocolate donut. They are both carbohydrate-based but obviously have very different effects in your body. The main point you need to remember is that you do need carbohydrates in your diet as it they are one of the three main macro-nutrients (with protein and lipids). You just need to know which ones to eat and which to avoid.

SUGAR

NATURAL - BETTER

Natural sugars exist in most plants to a variable degree, and also in dairy. When a sugar is in its natural form, it rarely threatens health, unless eaten in high volumes. The natural sugars from these clean whole foods, provide the body with its preferred source of energy, glucose.

Consider sources like apples, deeply coloured berries, citrus fruits, and also green beans, squash, leafy greens, sweet potatoes and most vegetables.

Dried fruits also offer plenty of natural, healthful sugars, however, they are highly concentrated versions of the original fruit, therefore, intensely sweet, so you must be aware to eat less of them.

Honey, unsulfured molasses, maple syrup, coconut nectar, fruit paste (dates, mashed bananas, apple sauce) are considered acceptable when used in moderation.

REFINED - POOR

When sugar is not naturally occurring in food, you should stay away from that food, or be warned and approach with caution.

Sugar cane is the tropical grass from which sugar comes. When you cut the stem of a sugar cane plant, a clear sweet liquid pours from it, just like maple water from the maple tree. This liquid is naturally refreshing and healthy because it has come from the plant and has not been refined by man as yet.

It is when this liquid is taken and refined in the multi-step process it takes to make refined sugar that you now have a dangerous ingredient. Stripped of the natural fibers of the cane plant and stripped of the nutrients that are in that plant, you are left with nothing more than a "bullet to the heart". You are left with a nutrient-dead substance that is also called a thief. The substance is so foreign to your body, that it doesn't recognize it nor does it know how to process it. In an effort to do something with it, your body is forced to take minerals from your organs and skeleton to neutralize this offensive substance, destroying and robbing you of your health. That is why refined sugar is a thief. It takes from the body, lessening your wellness.

Are all sugars bad? When you see the words 'raw cane sugar', 'brown sugar' and even 'agave,' you may be tempted to believe these are better options. Agave, once considered to be a healthy sugar alternative, has lost its healthy properties as it is now highly refined. None of these sweet options are of value to your health. It is important to be aware of the many manufacturing and marketing tricks at play in the sale of sugar.

THE IMPOSTERS – NO BETTER

There are numerous alternative sugars designed to give you the taste of sweet with the promise of not harming your body. The trouble is, they still trip the metabolic switches that launch the chemical processes in your organs of blood sugar handling that are required to mop up sugar. You are not getting a free ride. Stevia, aspartame, xylitol, high fructose corn syrup, sucralose, glucose, fructose, - hundreds of different names - are all sugar imposters. They have been designed to trick you into thinking you will be eating less sugar and that they are 'better' sweet options for you. But that isn't what happens. The organs of blood sugar handling – pancreas, liver, spleen, adrenals - are still called into action in response to these imposters. They are making you sick at dramatic rates. The fake sugar isn't helping.

Even worse, you are not making the connection mentally that you are consuming large amounts of sugar, refined or otherwise. It is much like feeding an addiction when you get hooked on sugar. In 1973, only two percent of the population in the United States had Type II Diabetes. It is to be noted that Type II Diabetes is a lifestyle disease. You are not born with it. You do it to yourself with your lifestyle choices and practices. A few decades later, nearly ten percent of the population has this once-rare disease and health care practitioners believe at least thirty percent of the population has undiagnosed Type II Diabetes or metabolic disorders. **The population has gone from eating 2 teaspoons of sugar a day, to 22.4 teaspoons per day!** The body can never handle that without disastrous consequences.

POP

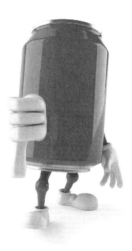

Pop is refined, liquid sugar. Period. Avoid it at all costs. Even the diet variety is of no benefit to you. Fruity sparkly beverages are no better. The average soda today contains ten teaspoons of sugar and each of these teaspoons contains 4 grams of sugar. One soda contains half the average amount of sugar North Americans consume. The Recommended Daily Allowance (RDA) of sugar advocated by the World Health Organization (WHO) is 6 grams per day. This number is readily met through consuming natural sugars in our diet and we rapidly exceed it in vast quantities by drinking even just one pop.

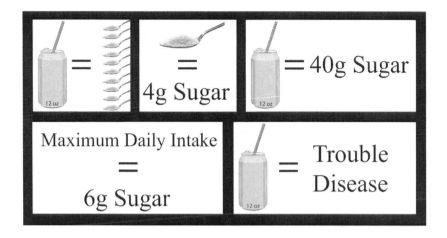

KEY CONCEPTS:

The only way to consume a grain is to prepare it properly by soaking it and souring it beforehand.

Fruit & vegetables are healthy carbohydrates.

Stay away from added sugar, any kind.

Run at the sight of pop.

CHAPTER 21:

MYTHS
PROTEINS

"Were the walls of our meat industry to become transparent, literally or even figuratively, we would not long continue to raise, kill, and eat animals the way we do."

— *Michael Pollan,*
The Omnivore's Dilemma: A Natural History
of Four Meals

MEAT

To eat meat or not to eat meat! There is a cultural shift in the eating of meat. Generally, less red meat is being consumed and when it is eaten, it is in smaller quantity. Vegetables are now taking centre stage on your plate in stark contrast to meat playing the starring role in past decades. Much of this is environmentally related as you challenge the nature in which meat has been produced. Meat has been linked to heart disease and cancer, higher rates of toxicity, numerous gastrointestinal infections because of bacteria in the food chain and other GI conditions. When livestock of any kind is in a concentrated feedlot, conditions conspire to make the animal sick. Animals are required to receive multiple pharmaceuticals containing heavy metals just to keep somewhat healthy. When you consume this meat, you are consuming whatever the animal ate, including heavy metals, pathogens, pharmaceuticals and other unknown agents.

Environmentally speaking, raising livestock accounts for fifteen percent of global greenhouse gas emissions every year. If cattle were a nation unto themselves, they would be the third highest producers of greenhouse gas emissions. Overconsumption of animal proteins imparts a high cost to human health. You only need fifty grams of protein per day, but most of you are getting sixty-eight grams, and in many places, ninety. You are witnessing an increased cost to healthcare and higher rates of most diseases, which is indirectly linked to meat consumption.

Today we are more mindful about meat and where it comes from. It is difficult to ignore that animals living in torturous conditions and then killed produced that piece of steak on your plate. More and more of you are choosing either not to eat meat or to eat less of it and when you do eat it, you choose to source it ethically.

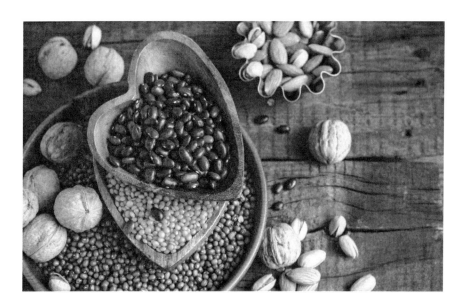

Hence the birth of meatless Mondays. Following a clean living lifestyle advocates eating well-sourced meats in moderation. The 'meatless Monday' concept should indeed happen more than once a week. More and more of you are opting for a vegetarian based lifestyle and whether or not you approach it as being strictly vegetarian, it can't be argued that everyone should eat more vegetables. Approach the consumption of meat with an eye to balance and consider adding more plant-based protein options to your clean living lifestyle.

POULTRY

If you are not eating organic poultry, you are unwittingly consuming a heavy dose of pharmaceuticals, antibiotics, heavy metals and other toxins. This is because the way poultry is raised today, in overcrowded 'chicken and turkey prisons' require numerous 'medicines' to keep the animals from dying. The flesh of these animals is tinged not only with poisons and toxins, but with negative energy. It bears consideration.

FISH

The same poor environment applies to fish. Concentration of mercury is so high in most oceanic fish and shell fish, in both wild and farm-raised, that you can only eat it so often. Toxins from the fish you consume will concentrate in your joints and muscles and central nervous system. That concentration will cause interrupted nervous system signaling causing erratic behavior, mental confusion, loss of balance, interrupt vision and illness in so many ways. If you consume fish and shellfish regularly, it is prudent to do a proper four-week cleanse at least twice per year. You can download Tosca's digital cleanse programs on line at www.toscareno.com.

You can't fool yourself into thinking that farm-raised fish is better for you. The same problems that effect poultry, effects farm raised fish. Typically, fish are kept in a "farm" in the water that closely resembles an underwater pen, where nothing is allowed in our out. Fish contained in that enclosure are swimming in each other's waste. It causes the fish to become unwell and therefore causes us to become unwell when we consume the flesh of these animals.

EGG

The egg has always been the gold standard for protein. Each egg contains four grams of protein and enough fat, of the right kind, to facilitate protein absorption. The egg white omelet, a 20th century concoction, is a mistake. Mother Nature in her infinite wisdom provided the ideal combination of nutrients in the egg to serve us best.

We were brainwashed to think that egg consumption caused high cholesterol. This is just not true. It is the massive consumption of sugar that causes this problem, as confirmed recently by the American and Canadian Hearth Association. The egg took the hit for something of which it was not guilty.

Eggs are an excellent source of well-rounded protein and if the birds that laid the eggs are well treated and fed as chickens like to be fed – grubs and bugs – then the egg is an ideal protein source for a clean living diet.

SOY

The reason soy was considered as a healthy food in first place was because in Okinawa, Japan, one of the Blue Zones*, the long-lived citizens consumed plenty of soy in the form of traditionally prepared tofu and miso. North Americans immediately jumped on the bandwagon and started eating soy. However, they were missing a crucial piece of information about the kind of soy the Okinawans were eating. Soy in Okinawa is non-GMO. Unfortunately, you and I don't have access to that kind of soy. Most of what you get is genetically modified (GMO) and chemically engineered and is best avoided.

Even though soy is a complete source of protein, the difficulty with soy is that it is a hormone-interrupter. All soy contains phytoestrogens, and these mimic naturally occurring phytoestrogens in the body. If you are a male eating soy, you may run the risk of developing more feminine characteristics than male. In women, the phytoestrogens in soy increase the chances of developing breast cancer. Soy competes for space with naturally occurring hormones in your body. It upsets the delicate and complex balance of hormones within you. Because you are all biologically unique, it would be hard to gauge what the effect of soy could be on your hormones. Soy is also contra-indicated with Hashimoto's Disease.

A further consideration about soy is that it is not usually ethically sourced as most of it comes from Asia where farming standards are lower. There is a very good chance that your soy has been exposed to pesticides, herbicides and other toxins, during the growing process. A final concern with soy is that it is highly genetically modified. The only good soy to consume is a fermented soy, in the form of tempeh, miso, natto, tamari.

QUINOA

Quinoa is NOT a grain. It is a seed that thinks it's a grain. Quinoa contains the highest amount of readily digestible protein of any plant. If you are a strict vegetarian or vegan, quinoa is your most valuable source of protein. It also happens to contain more calcium than an 8 oz glass of milk. Quinoa is extremely high in minerals and is versatile in the kitchen. It can be prepared savory or sweet.

Nathalie puts it in her daily salad and makes 'meat'-loaf, spaghetti sauce and meatballs with quinoa. Tosca makes morning breakfast cereals, breads, muffins and other baked goods using quinoa and often tops a green salad with it for plant-based protein.

The only caveat is that you must rinse quinoa seeds very well before cooking to remove the bitter coating. Quinoa comes from a plant that is a saponin, basically creating foam, suds and bitterness like soap. Make sure you rinse the grains thoroughly before cooking. Some people say: "I don't like the taste of quinoa". Maybe it is because you ate quinoa that had not been properly rinsed.

LEGUMES NUTS AND SEEDS

Manufacturers will use nut 'pieces' in making nut and seed butters. The problem with pieces of nuts and seeds is that as soon as they are opened and exposed to air, they begin to be negatively affected by oxygen and light. This causes rancidity. You don't realize when you buy chunky peanut butter that you are buying a product that may be rancid thanks to the nut or seed pieces used to make it.

Both Tosca and Nathalie make their own nut butters. Soak nuts and seeds first in order to remove the phytic acid found on all seeds. Removing this layer allows you to better access the nutrients within the nuts or seeds. What is phytic acid? All nuts, seeds and legumes sit in an envelope that contains the genetic information to create an entire plant. Phytic acid is that envelope that seals the nut or the seed shut until exposed to the right conditions to allow growth. The right conditions include light, soil and water. If you are going to consume any of these foods, you need to soak them first to access the nutrients properly. Phytic acid interferes with mineral absorption. Unless you soak away the phytic acid, you can't get to these minerals and it becomes a waste of money. That may be one of the reasons there are so many bone problems. If you can't access the minerals in foods like nuts, seeds and legumes, you cannot form strong bones in your body. Your forefathers consumed between four and forty times more minerals than you do today, where thus far more healthy.[8]

---

8   Weston A Price, Nutrition and Physical Degeneration.

KEFIR

Kefir is an ancient food. In the days before refrigeration, the story goes that the prophet Mohamed gifted the people of the Caucausus Mountains the secret of how to make this probiotic rich food. The people receiving the gift were told never to share the recipe because it imparted such health and vitality that they wanted to keep it for themselves. Kefir comes from the Turkish word KEIF which means 'feel good'.

Kefir is rich in taurine, tryptophan and other amino acids or proteins that have been naturally processed through fermentation to yield this miracle food. For a vegetarian or vegan, kefir is an important protein source especially when made with plant-based milk.

KEY CONCEPTS

Meat and poultry: If you are going to eat meat, make sure it is grass-fed and pasture-raised. Eat it in moderation.

Fish: Choose wild-caught and perform a thorough 4 week cleanse periodically.

Egg: A perfect protein. Eat the yolk too. Choose cage-free. Happy hens, happy eggs.

Soy: Make sure you are eatign soy that is non-GMO and properly prepared.

Quinoa: Complete plant-based protein. Make sure you rinse before cooking.

Legumes: Incomplete protein. Be sure to eat in combination with other ingredients to complete the protein profile such as rice and beans. Soak legumes before consuming.

Kefir: Amazing food. Beautiful and healthy probiotic food.

CHAPTER 22:

QUESTION YOUR ENVIRONMENT

"In a chronically leaking boat, energy devoted to changing vessels is more productive than energy devoted to patching leaks."

- Warren Buffett

Now that we have covered the three main macronutrients, you have many questions to answer about your environment.

Question: What in your environment supports your clean living?

Example:

I always have a bowl of fresh fruit on the counter and cut veggies in the fridge ready to eat in case I get hungry.

_____

Question: What in your environment needs to change?

Example:

I am very good at home, but when I eat out, I tend to surround myself with people who make very poor food choices.

I still think that diet soda is good for me or at least, not as bad.

Question: Who in your environment supports your best Self?

Example:

I feel good about myself whenever I hang out with my friend who exercises and eats well.

Question: What or who in your environment can help you identify what you need to work on?

Example:

My clothes don't fit me anymore and my body is a mess.

Question: What events happened in your past that could have influenced where you are now in your health? What changed in your life? Is there anything worth mentioning that could be linked to where you currently are?

Example:

I moved. I got a new job. I met someone. I got married. I got separated. I had a child. My kids moved away for school. I had a tragedy in my life. My father passed away.

Question: What is the relationship between these events and your current situation?

Example:

After I had my kids, I changed my priorities to serve the needs of my children and stopped focusing on myself.

Question: Think about the people in your environment, your parents, siblings, friends and/or partner. What is the relationship between these people (mother, father, brother, friend, etc.) and your current situation?

Example:

My mom always took me for ice cream when I was sad to make me feel better. She didn't know any better because that is what her mom used to do.

Question: What have I taught people around me about my tendencies or habits?

Example:

I am always the person people can count on as a drinking buddy, or to order dessert.

Question: Who will be with you once you have achieved your goal(s)?

Example:

I will be spending lots of time playing with my grandkids.

I will be surrounded by healthy and clean living people.

Question: What will no longer be in your environment when you reach your goal?

Example:

Junk and processed foods.

I will, somehow, happen to spend a lot less time with this friend who had a bad influence on me.

We will continue to encourage you to question other areas of your life throughout the book. By asking you to explore your environment, we have begun reprogramming the first of six of your neurological levels.

KEY CONCEPTS

Questioning yourself about your current situation helps you determine what you want.

Becoming aware of what surrounds you and who is in your environment are the first steps in re-training the brain to allow transformation to happen.

Going over the elements and people in your life that have affected your present situation is helpful to understand what led you to where you are now.

*"Nobody can go back and start a new
beginning, but anyone can start today and
make a new ending."*

- Maria Robinson

Now that you are aware of your environment and the myths about
the food present in our environment, we will move into the second
neurological level: BEHAVIOURS. Behaviours, our daily actions,
will be your best allies in your clean living journey. You will now
start to lay down the tracks of a new path where you choose and
adopt new and successful behaviours.

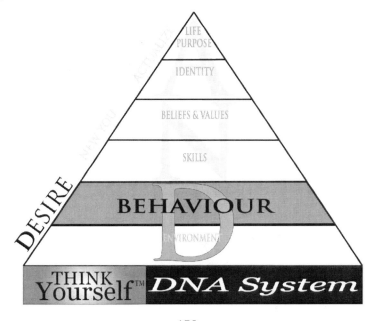

The Behaviour level includes your actions; what you do for a living, how you interact with those around you, your plans, and your successful or self- sabotaging behavioural choices.

This part is about the actions and choices you make. Our goal is to make your actions consistent with and supportive of what you want in your life. Luckily, you now know that the brain is malleable and that you are not stuck with a brain that has been conditioned to sabotage your success. You can rebuild your mental muscle and recondition your mind to create something beautiful and sustainable for yourself.

Question: What behaviour supports my clean living?

Example:

I spend time planning my meals for the week

Question: What behaviours need to change?

Example:

I eat take-out or stop at the drive-through because I leave it to the last minute when I am starving and make poor choices as a result.

We will now introduce a few questions which will require you to time-shift yourself in the future after having reached your goal. We will ask you about a time frame, evidence and proof of achieving that goal. For example, if your goal is to eat more plant-based food, you would say that you will have reached your goal when you are regularly buying fresh produce for your meals. You will think you are there when you are planning your meals, including lots of plant-based options and you are starting to crave plant-based goodness. You will also know it when you start to feel better than you have ever felt.

When do you want your outcome?

Decide on a realistic time frame in which to achieve your goal. What is your deadline? – Remember to time shift yourself in the future and phrase it in the present as if it had already happened.

Example:

It is March 2019 and I am now at my ideal weight. I am amazed at how simple the process was to change my habits and how easy it was to introduce more healthy choices that I now enjoy.

It is July 2019 and I am now at my ideal weight. I feel amazing with the empowering feeling of success that kicked in right away when I started this process.

I wanted to build a lean body with good muscle in a year, and I am almost there. It has been nearly a year and I am close to achieving my goal.

I am now in the process of achieving my ultimate goal of running a triathlon. It will happen step by step as I am dedicating time to make it happen.

What will you have accepted as evidence that you have achieved your outcome?

Example:

I am now smiling at myself in the mirror.

I have confidence in choosing clean options for me, there is no confusion anymore, I know what I need.

I am now smiling every time I think of what to make for dinner.

I am happy every day because I know how to take care of my body.

I am receiving recognition by my peers who want to know why my skin is so radiant and I have so much energy.

How do you know that reading this book has put you closer to your clean living?

What needs to happen when you finish reading that will prove to you that you attained something valuable?

Example:

I now have a clear vision of what my body and mind are capable of.

I feel a sense of general well-being.

I am setting up some time to work on my next goals.

I am free of my limiting beliefs and think differently about my cooking skills.

I now have a clear vision of what wellness means to me.

I now know how to advocate for myself and I use the book as a reminder.

What do you do now to 'feed' or nourish yourself?

Example:

I have signed up at a women's association and attend meetings on a regular basis to keep feeding myself with like-minded individuals.

What can you do now that you could not do before?

Example:

I am running my 5km weekly

I am wearing jeans 2 sizes smaller.

I go to my regular check-ups at the doctor and see an improved blood panel.

I can reduce or go off certain medications.

I can bend down and tie my own shoes easily.

Remember, you have to be able to personally do, authorize or arrange it. Anything outside your control is not 'well-formed'. Registering for a seminar is within your control. As is hiring a coach. Asking your employer for time off is not. The time off will only become well-formed if it is granted. For example, it is hard to predict that your family will also be happy with your changes. It would be a mistake to state that on paper, the same as it would be a mistake to predict the weather. Your well-formed outcome is about you and you have to be able to control it.

If your goal is to lose 220 lbs in a month, you might want to reconsider and put something more reasonably achievable in its place. It must be something that is humanly possible, and that you could potentially do. Your outcome has to be within the realm of human capability. If it is doable, then your brain can make you dream it and can make you right.

Is it achievable?

Example:

Yes, in fact, my neighbour has achieved clean living!

Yes, of course it is because there are many Facebook groups and organizations that support clean living so I know it is possible for me.

VISUALIZATION EXERCISE

We now invite you to do a mental exercise. As mentioned earlier, your unconscious mind can process over two million pieces of information every second. When you use your logic and write one answer, you more likely lose over a million of details, images, sounds, feelings that also came to mind as you were responding to the question. Remember that your brain can process information so much faster that you can write or express it on paper. Now take a moment to close your eyes and use your senses to add details. What will you see, hear and feel when you have your goal?

Make a mental image of your outcome. Include the details you need to make it more compelling. This question will be done in your head. See your outcome happening. See it as if it is happening now. Add more details based on your senses. What else do you see? What do you hear? What are you saying in your head? How do you feel? Place that image on a giant screen and turn up the dial. Add everything you need to make it nicer, brighter and more compelling. Dare to dream everything you want to be part of this picture. See yourself as a third person looking at yourself in the picture. Once you have seen everything you needed to see, heard everything you needed to hear and felt everything you needed to feel, take the picture and insert it in your timeline in your future. It is like placing the picture as a to-do list for your personal assistant. You are telling your unconscious mind that this is what will happen in your future. Your unconscious mind will keep working on achieving the result as it was just told that this was going to happen. Your brain doesn't know the difference between reality and fiction. It just executes your orders.

KEY CONCEPTS:

Aligning your behaviours with your goals lays down the foundation for sound serving habits.

Giving yourself deadlines and guidelines about what to look for when your goal will be achieved contributes to making your goals concrete and realistic.

Mentally rehearsing what you want, making your goal compelling using all senses will start making it real in your head.

CHAPTER 24:

CLEAN LIVING BEHAVIOURS

"It doesn't matter where you are; you are nowhere compared to where you can go."

- Bob Proctor

WELLNESS IS NOT A
ONE-SHOT DEAL

The average North American diet is unbalanced and decidedly unclean. Heavily skewed towards animal protein, processed and fried foods, high in sweets and lacking in fruits and vegetables, it is challenging to attain wellness based on this kind of eating. One clean meal will not solve a lifetime of poor eating.

What is important to understand is that it is nutrient imbalances that lead to weight gain. Eating Clean® solves weight problems not by diet but by solving nutrition problems. For example, an underactive thyroid is a common cause of slow metabolism. Increased stress levels and eating too much sugar triggers the release of stress hormones. There must be a lot of stress out there because the average North American diet consists of 18% sugar. When you consume sugar at the high rates of today, your body becomes low in the nutrient chromium. Sugar depletes the body of this mineral and others, as the body works to process it. This leaves you in an unbalanced and undernourished state. It is easy to see how illness happens.

The fix doesn't come from eating one big salad and calling it done. The fix is a long-term solution. It is a daily practice of a number of habits, layered one upon the other, building a wellness foundation from the inside out.

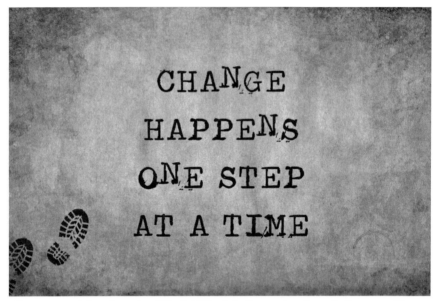

CHANGE HAPPENS ONE STEP AT A TIME

If you consider that the World Health Organization defines wellness as a combination of the three principles – Eating Clean®, Exercise and Emotional wellness – then it makes sense to implement these practices in your life. Eating is something you must do daily anyway, so learning how to Eat Clean® is a sound investment in your health. Exercise is a critical aspect of your wellness, so finding ways to move your physical self also matters. A moving, physically sound body is a well body.

While you know that Eating Clean® and Exercise are obvious elements of your Clean Living wellness strategy, it is not always clear that you must take care of your emotional self. In Traditional Chinese Medicine there is a saying that "if you don't take care of your emotions, your emotions will take care of you." This ancient wisdom suggests that emotions, if not dealt with, can destroy your health. By way of an example, the lung is the center for grief. For those who cannot express grief, the lung becomes a place where the emotions become stuck and diseases like lung cancer can result.

In the book, *Messages From the Body* by Narayan Singh, it is stated that, "physical symptoms arise from the condition of the individual's body as generated by negative thoughts the individual constantly has, that shape their life experiences through constant repetition." In other words, what you spend your time thinking about will become so. Leaving anger, guilt, resentment and fear inside the body, implants the seeds of disease.

Taking time to process how you feel and caring about how you feel, eases the dis-eased condition within the body. The practices of yoga, meditation and journaling offer a place to process emotion. Being at one with your physical body, learning to be present in it and with it, helps to shed the burdens you carry. Science proves that meditating for a mere 10 minutes per day, dramatically alters the blood chemistry, reducing levels of stress hormones in the blood. Those short 10 minutes (which you may feel you don't have time for) can literally save your life.

The same is true for the practice of giving thanks. When you acknowledge the goodness in your life you simultaneously acknowledge the presence of a power greater than yourself. To be humbled, to give thanks, despite your circumstances, sparks an energy that brings you closer to your true self. Giving thanks is the quickest way to improve your mood or vibrational energy. Spend some time giving thanks each day. Practicing gratitude profoundly shifts your attitude and your wellness.

Finally, you can help to process your thoughts, feelings, ideas and gratitude by journaling. The act of committing thought to paper cements that thought, confirming it to be, deeply within the brain. It is a powerful way to process your emotional self when you commit thought to paper. Writing de-clutters your mind, helping you process. Writing helps you gain a bank of knowledge. Writing helps you bear witness to your own growth. Writing helps you make sense of your own life. Writing boosts your chance for success in all you endeavor by as much as 50%. All of these combined to enhance your wellness.

You may wonder what the traits and habits of a person who follows a clean lifestyle are. What does he or she do to keep the body lean and the mind healthy? After 17 years working in the fitness and wellness industry, Tosca has observed the practices of clean people and can deliver the following set of observations.

COMMON CLEAN LIVING PRACTICES

Clean living people:

- Do not count calories.

- Do not body shame or judge.

- Recognize that every meal is an opportunity to nourish the body.

- Source their foods responsibly to the best of their ability.

- Prepare their foods properly, often using traditional preparation techniques.

- Seek to nourish rather than diet.

- Do not feel as if they are making sacrifices when they cannot eat junk.

- Use a journal to record their progress and their emotional journey.

- Do not obsess about one or two meals that are not completely clean. They eat and behave in moderation and in balance.

- Choose to follow the Eat Clean® lifestyle out of free will.

- Clean Living people understand that they have agency over their wellness decisions and self-care practices.

- Drink 3 liters of water per day, or more if very active.

- Eat 5 – 6 smaller meals per day, spaced 2 – 4 hours apart.

- Base every meal on a proper balance of protein, carbs and fat:

- 30% fat + 30% protein + 40% carbohydrates (20% greens + 20% fruits, dairy and grains) = Macronutrient Balance

- Avoid refined, processed foods.

- Stop eating after 8:00 pm in the evening.

- Pack a cooler filled with clean foods to get through the day.

- Prepare nuts, seeds and grains by soaking them first.

- Eat grass fed, organic meats as much as possible.

- Include plant protein in their diet along with animal protein and bone broth.

- Often have a lean healthy body weight.

- Pursue physical activity for the joy of it.

- Practice gratitude on a daily basis.

- Do not skip meals to manage their weight.

- Never skip breakfast.

- Don't count calories.

CLEAN LIVING LESSONS

Now we will share some Clean Living Success Stories to give you an idea of how powerful and practical this lifestyle is.

Ed

Several years ago, Ed began to pop up on my social media platforms. Obese and weighing over 300 pounds, Ed was frustrated by the never-ending promises of fad diets. Nothing was working for him. Every diet he tried just made him gain more weight. Finally, a friend told him about the Eat Clean Diet®. That friend encouraged Ed to try it because it wasn't about counting calories or starving. It was about eating correctly. Over the course of two years, Ed made stunning progress. He stopped drinking coffee with triple, triple sugar and cream. He started drinking more water. He exchanged the boxed and prepackaged foods he had been eating for colourful, fresh produce and plenty of lean meats. When he added exercise to his new wellness habits, like magic, his whole body changed. He was now the proud owner of a lean, muscular physique and had loads of sparkling energy to spare. He was a new man. Now he is a fitness instructor and runs marathons!!

Brenda and Dawn, Mother and Daughter

After years of struggling to gain healthy weight, Brenda, mother to Dawn, found success by Eating Clean®. Dawn had an eating disorder and was dangerously underweight, so much so that she was hospitalized. Brenda gave Dawn a copy of the Eat Clean Diet® and in it, her daughter found the permission she needed to eat smaller meals more frequently. Dawn was released from hospital and was soon gaining weight at a steady and healthy pace. Mother and daughter signed up for yoga classes and began to meditate on a daily basis. The process of returning to health through clean living was long and slow but what was stunning was that it stuck. Where all the other diets only served to worsen the situation, Eating Clean® stuck. Both Brenda and Dawn are living in optimal wellness today, feeling blessed with a second chance. They eat clean, healthy foods to serve their wellness, and they do it with joy.

Sam Adams

Sam was frustrated with her efforts to lose weight and exercise. She wanted to lose 30 pounds and see some definition in her body. She wanted to get rid of her meno-pot. Initially she felt her diet was good. At 52 she had run a few half marathons and felt pretty good. But then there were times that she wanted to eat everything in sight. She had had enough. She started to follow the Eat Clean® lifestyle by first ridding her body of refined sugar and sugar products by doing Tosca Reno's 4-week Strike Sugar program. The biggest change she made was to remove soda from her diet – she was drinking several Cokes a day – and exchanged it for water. She lost 12 pounds very quickly and those results encouraged her to continue with the lifestyle. In a few months Sam had lost the 30 pounds she had wanted to and discovered new levels of energy. She felt like life was good again.

KEY CONCEPTS:

Wellness is an on-going journey.

By committing to clean living practices, you slowly pave your new road to wellness.

CHAPTER 25:

YOUR POSITIVE OUTCOME

"A year from now you will wish you had started today."

- Karen Lamb

It is now time to write the software that will reprogram your brain to make the jump into a more successful arena. You can use a recap of everything you discovered in the previous exercises to write down the perfect clean life scenario in the context you are considering. State what you want in positive terms. i.e. What do you want? Where do you want it? When do you want it? Example: "I want to be, do or have X". If the answer forms as "I do not want..." then ask yourself: "What do I want instead of..." If it feels totally untrue when you say it out loud, you may want to start your statement with: ''I am willing to learn how it feels to be clean," giving yourself permission to evolve. You also want to avoid the xx-Free type of statement. i.e. I want to be stress-free, debt-free, etc. These are toxic words and need to be re-phrased positively.

Examples:

My name is... and I am feeling happy in my kitchen. It makes me happy to prepare clean, fresh food for my family for every meal. I no longer have fear about making meals. I am always fully prepared and ready. I am happy to create new clean meals that serve my family well and I see the results. My children are happier and healthier, and my husband and

I don't argue about little things. I am loving my new schedule of taking the time to enjoy the evening meal every day with them.

My name is... and I am feeling great in my skin. I love moving my body every day, and I feel energized all day long. I feel strong and capable. I have developed meal planning skills that enabled me to make clean food choices, a habit that is second nature to me now.

Example of someone whose daughter's wedding is coming up:

My name is ………. and I am looking fabulous and feeling wonderful in my mother-of-the-bride's dress that I am wearing at my daughter's wedding this summer. I learned about clean living and implemented the principles, so I could enjoy my daughter's wedding without feeling ashamed. My new healthy body makes me happy and promotes a sense of well-being I have not had in a long time. People are telling me how fabulous I look. I feel proud and happy to have had the energy and clarity of mind to be involved in the planning. I can see myself enjoying the warm summer day of the wedding and can smell the scents of the flowers in the air. I have a wonderful feeling going through my body that will keep me happy for years to come.

My name is.... and I am in control of my wellness. I love that I have a newfound energy and confidence in my body and my abilities. I now feel full to bursting with potential and with energy. I have time to exercise and eat well and I am in the best shape of my life. I hear people tell me how great I look, and I feel amazing. I love myself.

My name is.... and I love my new life. I have successfully changed my old behaviours into new clean living habits that are serving me well. I can get through every day in an optimistic and happy way. and I have the self-confidence to introduce myself to highly intelligent, attractive and motivated people like me. I am happy to be surrounded by positive influences that keep me on track with my new choices. I always find ways to stay motivated and inspired.

Your turn, write your positive outcome:

My name is _____ and I _____

_____

_____

_____

_____

_____

_____

Once you have written your outcome, place copies of this statement all over your house, in every room and in your car. Write everything as if it's happening in the present, as if it's happening right now. Record yourself saying it out loud at least 10 times and play the recording every morning and every night.

You can add to your statement as time goes by. It is always good to keep it updated and make sure that your statement changes and evolves with you and your changing desires. Listen to this statement several times a day and at least ten times out loud so that your brain hears it out loud. There is a popular belief that it takes 21 days to re-create new neural pathways through the brain, to create the new habit. This statement came from Doctor Maxwell Maltz in the 1950s from research with patients that were receiving plastic surgery. It would take them, on average, 21 days to get used to their new nose, for example.[9]

As you now realize, this research, although quite popular, is dated. I prefer to follow the results of Doctor Phillippa Lally who conducted research in 2009 with volunteers who chose an eating, drinking or activity behaviour to carry out daily, in the same context for 12 weeks. The study published in the European Journal of Social Psychology reported that the average time to reach automaticity for performing an initially new behaviour, was 66 days.[10] That's quite a big difference from 21!

Read it for at least 2 months (66 days). If you catch yourself thinking negative thoughts, turn them into positive thoughts. It took years for you to get where you are now, it might take a few months to reset your brain and create new habits. Be patient with yourself. It is a journey.

---

9   http://www.jamesclear.com/new-habit
10   http://www.ucl.ac.uk/news/news-articles/0908/09080401

KEY CONCEPTS:

Use every thought you have generated so far to write down a positive outcome that will satisfy your desires.

Once you have elicited your outcome, continue to read it and keep letting your brain know that this is what you want.

Knowing what you want and writing your expectations & desires will set the tone for the unconscious mind to open the gate to new possibilities.

CHAPTER 26:

THE RETICULAR ACTIVATING SYSTEM

"Don't focus on what you DON'T want.
The reticular activation system of the brain
is really, really good at what it does--if
you unwittingly tell it to go searching for
trouble, heartache, or disappointment, it will
absolutely find it, guaranteed, every time."

- John Assaraf

We are about to start clearing your brain to make room for your new outcome in the NEW YOU section of the D.N.A. System. We will also anchor your positive outcome in the ACTUALIZE section. What you have done so far was to tell your brain what you DESIRE.

As you go through the next steps of the System, continue to read and listen to your outcome many times per day. This will help your brain become well wired and well programmed to always continue working on it, whether you are conscious of it or not. You know how sometimes you think about a song and you just cannot remember the title of the song? Then you stop thinking about it and it comes back two hours later? Although you think you stopped thinking about it, your brain (your personal assistant) kept working on it. It never stopped looking for the title as you had ordered it to do when you said: "I will remember it later." A brain that is well wired will always deliver and follow your ultimate order without being distracted by irrelevant or unimportant things.

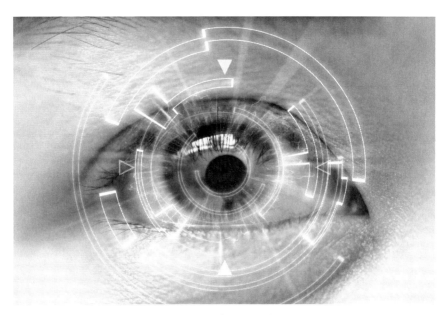

Here is a concrete example of how a brain that is programmed for something will follow the ultimate goal as opposed to being distracted by a short-term gain. Nathalie, who thinks that she is the luckiest person in the world and that she always gets what she wants, tells the story: ''A few years ago we were in Mexico with a group. Our friends were going to a restaurant one evening. They had made a reservation for 10. We wanted to join them, so we tried to get the reservation changed to 12 and even though I used my Spanish to negotiate with the waiter, nothing worked! I was just not able to convince him. Somehow, I was losing my Spanish, and the words were not coming easily. They said they could not accommodate 12 of us. My husband and I had to eat somewhere else that night. I went to a thirty-second loop of disappointment and then turned things around and had a fabulous romantic dinner just the two of us. I thought it was impossible. How could this be happening? I always get what I want! The day after, at the hotel, all ten of our friends were sick with food poisoning.''

THE RETICULAR ACTIVATING SYSTEM.

You have a very small part of your brain called the Reticular Activating System (RAS). The RAS pays attention both to your environment, as well as to where you tend to place your attention (needs, wants, desires). It is always assessing and discerning what is relevant and important, in order to keep you safe AND help to get you what you want.

In the example above, Nathalie, who has programmed her brain to be safe and healthy, somehow must have picked up something she was not aware of. Maybe she glanced through the kitchen at the restaurant and her unconscious mind noticed that the meat was stored on the counter and not in the fridge. Maybe one of the two million things she overheard with her unconscious mind, as she was walking to the restaurant, was someone saying they had been sick eating there before, or it could have been anything. Nathalie's RAS protected her from being sick.

There you have it! If you are well programmed, you don't need to think about it anymore. Your brain works for you and makes things happen for you. Even if you don't see it right away.

Some people call it the Universe, some people call it God. Everybody has a different name for when these things happen. We just like to think that these instances are just another example of how powerful the brain is.

KEY CONCEPTS:

THE RETICULAR ACTIVATING SYSTEM

The RAS pays attention both to your environment, as well as to where you tend to place your attention (needs, wants, desires). It is always assessing and discerning what is relevant and essential, to keep you safe AND help get you what you want.

PART 6

THE "N"

CHAPTER 27:

NEW YOU

"Never too old, never too bad, never too late, never too sick to start from scratch once again."

- Bikram Choudhury.

Now that you have completed the D part of the D.N.A. System, you know who you are and what you want. In the NEW YOU section, you'll be introduced to a cleanup phase, necessary before installing your desires.

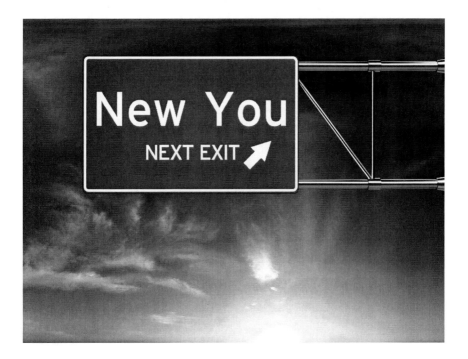

We will now study the next two layers of your brain. The Skills and Beliefs and Values levels will allow you to unravel deeper layers of yourself through questions, processes and exercises.

You will find out how you create your model of reality. Sometimes you imagine constraints and barriers that do not exist. They may just be in your head. You will discover how to turn the negative into positive and how to change your nemesis into a NEW YOU by neutralizing the past.

The second step of the D.N.A. System is to make room to implement what you just elicited. Your unconscious mind has already started to work on your desires. Your outcome has been planted and now you need to make sure that there is plenty of space for your outcome to grow. Just like in our original example, in order to get the new dream kitchen, you need to do demolish and remove what no longer works, including the out-dated cupboards. When you are planning a kitchen renovation, you will create a folder where you will file samples of the cupboards to match the backsplash, the tile, paint colours, granite for the countertop, hardware samples and so on. This is what you have just done in your brain. You have just made your folder and filled it with what you want. However, the reality is: it is just a folder. It is not a new kitchen. You cannot cook and entertain people in that folder. There is still much work to be done in order to realize your new kitchen.

Many books end after this creative folder has been made. THINK Yourself® CLEAN continues and guides you to the next steps to concretize your dream.

Rest assured that every method used in this book is light and effortless. When working with a new client, Nathalie sometime can sense their stress level rising when she mentions this part. They think that she will psychoanalyze their past and they will have to re-live their negative experiences and dig through the dirt, crying and suffering until the demons have been exorcised. Please. Relax. You are not about to do any of this. This is the best part. The clearing section is empowering, insightful, cleansing and most of all, fun and easy!

KEY CONCEPTS:

NEW YOU

You have elicited your desire and now is time to make room in order for your outcome to have space to be implemented

CHAPTER 28

SKILLS

*"Each person's task in life is to become an
increasingly better person."*

- Leo Tolstoy.

The third neurological level, Skills and Capabilities, makes us
realize what you are good at. What comes to you "naturally".

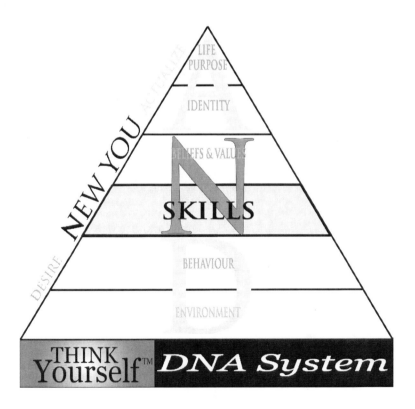

From a neuroscience perspective, you are starting to soften and disengage the old neural pathways. It is imperative at this point that you rewire. And so, begins the very exciting process of reinvention!

You are now invited to embrace your unique strengths and simultaneously unravel and disengage from impairments to your growth and progress. Stay the course to your greatest success. The skills questions below, will guide you through discovering and refining them.

Write down what you do very well. These are the skills you do effortlessly. Think of the things people say about you when they are astonished with your talent or your finished product: "I don't know how you do it! There is no way I could do this." That means it is a skill. Everybody can brush their teeth, which is a behaviour, but not everybody can remember the words of all the songs they hear. That is a skill.

What skills come easily and are effortless for you? Name some things you do well:

Example:

I can make any recipe from scratch.

I can create delicious meals with just a few clean ingredients.

I am disciplined when it comes to planning my workouts.

How do you feel strong? Alive? In charge?

Example:

I feel so much satisfaction from whipping up a meal quickly, in minutes. I got this!

Do you have, or can you obtain the resources, both tangible and intangible that you need to achieve your outcome? Resources include knowledge, beliefs, objects, premises, people, money and time. Do you need to read more books on your specific domain? Do you need to subscribe to podcasts or mindset websites or blogs that will feed you with information during your success journey? Do you need to hire a life coach who will create a specific program for you and help you stay on track?

Do you have all the resources you need to achieve your outcome?

Example:

Yes, I do, I have been reading so many books, registered to so many seminars, now I realize that it is all inside of me.

I will hire a coach who will walk with me through the path towards my new life.

What do you want or need to learn or get better at?

Example:

I need to learn how to prepare clean foods correctly.

I need to know how to balance my macronutrients to create a clean, healthy meal that nourishes me properly.

I need to learn how to read food labels.

I need to learn better culinary skills.

I want to be better at locating sustainable clean food in my area.

Where are you edging towards taking greater risks?

Example:

I need to get out of my comfort zone when it comes to trying new recipes.

In which ways do you now trust yourself that you did not before?

Example:

In looking at my 'have-done it' list, I realize how much I have grown in the past year.

I would always ask a friend to come to the gym with me because I was too scared to go on my own. Now I know how to use the equipment in the gym and feel I belong there. I am confident in my abilities to train correctly.

I am now so much better at selecting clean food when I grocery shop.

Now that you have defined what you want in the DESIRE section and equipped yourself with knowledge about your skills, you are able to cross the bridge between what you want and how to make the changes in your head in order for your unconscious mind to move in the same direction.

With the knowledge you gained from responding to the questions and learning about the technique to which you were just introduced, you now feel more powerful after the culmination of work from the first three levels. You are starting to get out of your way and embrace the best parts of yourself. It is beginning to feel possible to have a new and joyful life.

KEY CONCEPTS:

SKILLS

Skills are truly about acknowledging your gifts and strengths and trusting yourself to make empowered choices from this moment forward.

CHAPTER 29:

CONCRETE SKILLS

"If opportunity doesn't knock, build a door."

- Milton Berle

If you are looking for more skills to add to your toolbox, Tosca and Nathalie have already published multiple books on specifics about clean living.

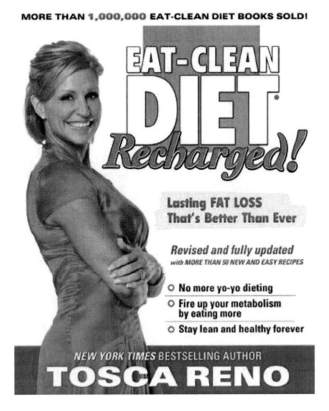

Tosca wrote The Eat Clean® Diet Recharged, the first book written on the subject when everyone else was giving us recipes or ways to eat clean, Tosca kicked off the eat clean revolution by modelling and teaching a holistic lifestyle that she first applied on herself to heal herself and transform her life. It is a complete mind-body and spiritual approach to restoring wellness.

For more on Tosca's book visit:

https://toscareno.store/collections/books

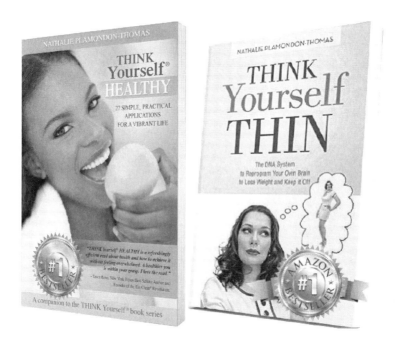

To learn more on weight loss, you can read Nathalie's books THINK Yourself® THIN and THINK Yourself® HEALTHY, teaching you practical applications of techniques you can focus on your health in your everyday life. www.thinkyourself.com

CHAPTER 30

BELIEFS & VALUES

"Your Beliefs are a magnet that creates your reality."

- Coach Bobbi

Your model of reality is created from your beliefs and values. At the Beliefs and Values level, you discover how to replace the old cupboards with the new ones. There is no room in your kitchen to keep them all - old and new ones. You need to remove the unwanted limiting beliefs and create more space for the new beliefs to take root.

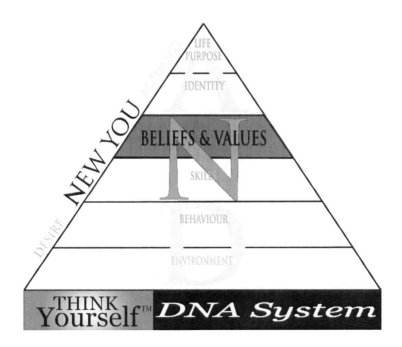

We will teach you how to put your model of reality to service and change that model of reality to better suit your goals of clean living. If you live in a model that says that you are clean and healthy, you will suddenly start noticing the opportunities to thrive, instead of finding excuses. You will be spending more time building long-lasting habits and not even think about junk food and skipping your workout. Allow your unconscious mind to do the necessary tweaking that will serve you even better. To do that, you need to work on the beliefs and value level.

The following questions will teach you how to identify what is important to you. What you believe to be true. What you value. What you would defend. What you used to perceive as your limitations, your weaknesses, your boundaries and mostly your potential.

You will discover that you can be whatever you want to be. This section will help you shake the box so that you can get out of it. It is like taking a crow bar and lifting the old counter top off so that it is easier to remove. It will soften your limits and help you see yourself from within as opposed to seeing yourself from the outside, looking at your limitations.

What do you consider sacred?

Example:

My body.

My health.

What do you value most?

Example:

My family

Health and wellness

Having fun in everything I do

What have you been afraid to look at?

Example:

I have been afraid at looking at my fitness level and my ability to perform simple everyday tasks.

I have been avoiding this high blood pressure condition, for years now, and I have been afraid to face it and learn why I feel so unwell.

What do you want to let go of that you feel is holding you back?

Example:

I want to let go of my poor eating habits and my fear of not knowing what I would be eating in a clean lifestyle.

What will come into your life that's currently missing?

Example:

I will have more self-confidence.

I will have better relationships.

I will have energy to run with my dog.

I will feel amazing as I lose the weight I gained when I had kids.

Where in your life do you find yourself doing the opposite of what you want to be doing, or know you should be doing, to support your clean living?

Example:

Often after lunch, I have to run an errand or do a delivery. En route, I go through the coffee shop drive-thru and grab a Caramel Explosion coffee with whipped cream and a S'mores cookie to go with it. This leaves me feeling (a) temporarily comforted ... which is quickly followed by (b) disgust at my lack of self-control. I KNOW it is the wrong choice. Emotionally, it leaves me feeling out of control, it ruins the healthy dinner I had planned for later, and I have noticed my skin is breaking out and my pants are becoming a bit snug.

The next few questions will open your unconscious mind, allowing you to dig deeper. They are being asked in opposite affirmations or negations to force your unconscious mind to dig for different answers. They are the Cartesian coordinates of the brain. Have fun with them and pay attention to the nuances in the questions. Remember that your unconscious mind loves that stuff. This could be the section that makes you generate the light bulbs you need to drive yourself to your outcome.

What will happen if you get it?

Example:

I will be happy with myself.

What won't happen if you get it?

Example:

I won't be ashamed of myself anymore.

What will happen if you don't get it?

Example:

I will continue feeling depressed and unhappy.

What won't happen if you don't get it?

Example:

I will never know how it feels to be well again.

The next six questions are an overview of the beliefs and values questions we have asked so far. In light of your previous answers, you will be amazed at how quickly you will find answers to this last series of questions.

CORE question: What do you believe you are and will always be?

Something you are, at your core, you are happy to be that way, as you want to be like that, and you know in your core that you will always be it. What are you proud and content to be?

Example: Caring.

POTENTIAL question: What is something you want to be and believe you could become?

Something you are hoping to become. Something you are excited about becoming.

Example: Organized at meal planning.

LIMITATION question: What is something you want to be but believe you are not?

Something you see as your limit? You would like to be that way, but you feel trapped and frustrated as you don't seem to be able to be it.

Example: Slim and fit.

BOUNDARY question: What is something you don't want to be and never will be?

You don't want to be that way, and you feel very strongly about never becoming that way either. What is off limits? What is your boundary? You don't ever want to be that way.

Example: I don't want to be starving myself in an effort to get well.

WEAKNESS question: What is something you don't want to be but believe you could become?

What is your weakness or your defect? Are you afraid you might become this? This may cause you anxiety as you don't want to be that way and you may become it.

> *Example: I am afraid I could become sick from eating so much junk food.*

SHADOW question: What is something you don't want to be, but you are afraid you are?

Something you feel guilty about, or of that which you are ashamed.

> *Example: I am afraid I am lazy.*

In light of all the questions you have responded to in this chapter, take a moment to reflect on what resonates as something from this exercise that you will be interested in exploring later. Ask yourself what was your 'aha' moment? What is the golden nugget of this chapter? Remember which beliefs and values will be the saviour of your shadow.

You now have a different view of yourself. You have opened up your mental process and set up a path favourable to assist with your transformation. You have just pulled the old cupboards from the wall with a crowbar and now it will be much easier to remove them and get rid of them. Negative limits, shadows, weaknesses, defects or boundaries have been loosened up and are ready to leave your body. This is what we will do in the next chapter.

KEY CONCEPTS:

BELIEFS & VALUES

You have your own model of reality, and when you operate within your model, you are always right.

Facing questions bravely will put you back in control, rather than being driven by your subconscious mind's limiting beliefs.

Understanding what you believe and what is important to you is the fuel that will continue to drive you towards clean living.

Using your core and your potential is the key to shifting your limitations and boundaries. Once identified, you know in which area of your life you may hold negative, limiting beliefs. When you choose to pay attention to these limiting beliefs, and banish them, you can let go of your weaknesses and shadows and transform yourself to what you really want to be.

CHAPTER 31:

NEGATIVE TO POSITIVE

"To create more positive results in your life,
replace "if only" with "next time.""

- Celestine Chua

You have learned, in the Neurological levels section, how beliefs and values are crucial and how they can affect your behaviour. The problem occurs when these beliefs are negative. These are called limiting beliefs.

Nathalie uses specific processes when she works one-on-one with her clients to clear negative emotions and limiting beliefs from their mind. These processes are not ideal to explain in a written form. That is why we have created this section to help you transform your limiting beliefs using a Question and Answers format.

We have also created the THINK Yourself® CLEAN video series which guides you through all the processes, questions and activities mentioned in this book. You can subscribe to the video series to access recordings which will help with a deeper cleaning.

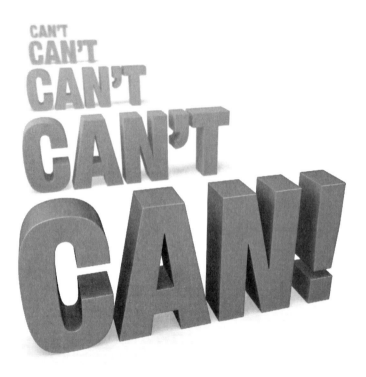

You will now turn Negative into Positive. The questions below are part of a process that will open up the boundaries of your unconscious limits. When you are in a problem box, sometimes you don't realize it. The following exercise will open windows and tear down walls so you can see outside the box. The resulting realizations will generate the light bulbs in your head that will help you let go of your old beliefs. It will make you recognize that these beliefs that you thought were part of your life are only real in your head and are not serving you. Therefore, they must go.

The power of words is potent and the study of the use of words is called linguistics. You can break down and solve any problem linguistically. Words impact your behaviours. Remember the expression, "whether you think you can or think you can't, you are always right." You will start noticing your thoughts and be able to mentally hit the Cancel button whenever you get a negative thought. You will catch yourself having a negative thought and replacing it with a good thought.

You can start with a question that is so common you may not think is a big deal. Since you are faced with this question multiple times daily, it is imperative to learn how to alter your response. When people ask you: "How are you doing?" Create your new response. Use positive words to create your situation. Think about it the next time you are about to respond with the usual "I'm okay, thank you." *Okay*? That's it? That is your total aspiration? With the word *okay,* you just told your brain that you want to be *okay and nothing more.* Consider this answer: "Not too bad". That is even worse. You now know that your personal assistant hears: "bad" and puts that on your list. Take this opportunity and every time someone asks you how you're doing to say instead: "I am fabulous", "I am awesome", "I am fantastic"? The power of these positive words will serve you well when programming your brain to be amazing!

Consider the anticipation of a negative feeling that has not happened yet, but you plan ahead to feel bad about anyway. Nathalie once asked the simple question: *"How are you?"* to a client. Nathalie tells the story:

"When I asked my client, "How are you?" she said: "I am tired! Well, I am not tired now, but I will be by the end of the day. I have so much to do! I have to pick up the kids after work and take one to soccer, another to guitar lessons and I will probably get stuck in traffic and get upset."

I asked: "Are you tired now?" She said: "No, not yet." "Are you in traffic now?" I asked. She said: "No not yet." I said: "Why are you already programming yourself to be tired and upset? Why aren't you saying instead: "I will feel wonderful tonight because I will have accomplished so much in my day. I will take advantage of the traffic to catch up on listening to my audio book. It will be awesome! Also, while my son is at soccer, I will drop my daughter off at her guitar lessons and take 20 minutes to go for a short run to energize myself before I pick them up again at the end of their sessions."

Do you have a global positioning system – GPS? Does it kick in when you get off track and decide to turn when it is not time? What does you GPS say? *Recalculating*! Every time you get off track, use the verbal cue *"recalculating"* to return to your correct position. When you hear yourself say: "I am so overweight!" Quickly hear yourself say: "Oh, wait, what did I just think? *Recalculating*! I am in the process of getting back in shape." Tosca frequently says, "cancel, clear, delete" when a negative message pops into her brain.

Here is your chance to start to *recalculate* more of your thoughts. The next series of questions will require you to dig deeper to uncover what has been keeping you from reaching your goals. What beliefs do you hold that could be transformed to serve you better? You are the result of what you think and what you have been thinking your entire life.

How do you feel about clean living?

> *Example:*

> *I am afraid that eating clean means that I have to give up all the things I love.*

What is your belief about it? Does it have to be hard?

Example:

I believe that clean living cannot happen without having to spend a lot of money and time changing every item in my kitchen.

I believe eating clean is expensive and complicated and doesn't taste good.

How can you change these beliefs?

Example:

With a bit of planning, I can choose clean recipes that allow me to slowly phase out less nutritious foods. In time I will have a clean kitchen and feel more in alignment with healthy living.

I am willing to learn and experiment with new food and learn how to prepare them so that they taste amazing.

Do you believe you'll ever adopt a clean lifestyle?

Example:

I have been dreaming about feeling well and looking amazing for so long that I think I am now used to it being just a dream, somewhere really far in some potential future. I fear that it may just always stay in the future.

How can you change this belief?

Example:

I am willing to re-program my beliefs so that I can break down my big dream into realistic and concrete steps. Each small step will bring me closer to achieving it.

In light of the answers to these questions about your beliefs about CLEAN LIVING, you may now realize how your language and thoughts shift your mindset and allow you to succeed.

Your success begins with your thoughts. Thoughts become actions and actions become habits. The philosopher Lao Tzu said:

> *Watch your thoughts; they become words.*
> *Watch your words; they become actions.*
> *Watch your actions; they become habits.*
> *Watch your habits; they become character.*
> *Watch your character; it becomes your destiny.*

USE YOUR SENSES TO RE-WRITE LIMITING BELIEFS

There are many ways to enhance your language. Use your senses when you re-phrase them. Make it happen in your head with visual, auditory and sensory details. What will happen when you start believing these things? You're going to *see* yourself getting up to prepare a clean breakfast. You will feel refreshed and vibrant, ready to take on the day as a result. You will *hear* yourself talking with confidence about how well you now sleep, how much energy you have and how your mood has improved. You will *see* yourself working out, lifting weights and being active. You will *hear* the voice inside your head telling you how wonderful it is to move your body with joy and excitement every day. You will *trust* that you understand and love clean living. That you are awesome! How are you going to *feel* when you can say, "*I love my new sense of wellness*"? Sentences that include senses and emotions are powerful.

Here are the limiting beliefs we had identified when we introduced the Beliefs and Values level in Part 4 of this book. Let's have a second look at them and see how they can be re-phrased.

EATING CLEAN IS HARD.

Depending on where you are with your mind shifting, you can re-phrase from one extreme to the other. You could choose to re-phrase this way:

> *Example Re-phrase:*
>
> *Being successful at clean living is easy.*

Which may be really pushing it depending on where you are at this time. You may want to choose a more transitional language like:

> *Example Re-phrase:*
>
> *I am learning how it feels to be successful at clean living. Already, I feel better.*
>
> *This time it will be different. I know I used to think clean living was challenging and that is the reason why I thought it was hard because I had chosen to think it was. Now that I am seeing it as easy as I practice more and implement small clean living steps, I will succeed easily.*

Here are more examples of re-phrasing the limiting beliefs introduced in Part Four:

BEING HEALTHY IS HARD.

> *Example Re-phrase:*
>
> *Being healthy is easy when we follow a clean living plan.*

Being healthy is rewarding.

EATING CLEAN IS EXPENSIVE

Example Re-phrase:

Being sick is more expensive and highly inconvenient.

Clean food is more nutrient dense, so you don't need as much of them.

IN MY FAMILY, WE WERE TOLD THAT A GOOD MEAL NEEDED TO INCLUDE MEAT, STARCHES, SAUCES AND DESSERT.

Example Re-phrase:

A good meal means a combination of macronutrients that includes fats, proteins and complex carbohydrates.

A well balanced, clean meal imparts a feeling of well-being.

THAT IS HOW I AM; I AM DOOMED TO STAY THIS WAY.

Example Re-phrase:

The body is a complete textbook of what we have done to it, and it can be remodeled at any age.

I am the person that I choose to be.

NO DIET WORKS FOR ME. NO MATTER WHAT I DO, I CAN'T LOSE WEIGHT.

Example Re-phrase:

A clean living lifestyle will work for me.

I have changed my limiting beliefs, and I now know that I am in the process of reaching my ideal weight.

I DON'T HAVE WILL POWER, SO I CAN'T STOP EATING SUGAR, SALTY, CRUNCHY, WINE AND CHOCOLATE.

Example Re-phrase:

Education helps me understand why I was drawn to these foods; now I am developing a healthy control over my choices.

I am in the process of becoming a strong advocate for my wellness.

EATING CLEAN® IS A LOT OF WORK.

Example Re-phrase:

Eating clean becomes easier the more I do it and the better I am at knowing what is healthy for me.

I can learn anything.

I HAVE CHILDREN SO I CANNOT EAT CLEAN®.

Example Re-phrase:

Eating clean is beneficial for all ages and stage of life.

My children are the reason I want to eat clean, so they motivate me to keep going.

What are your limiting beliefs?

1.

2.

3.

4.

5.

Use your words – linguistic skills - to re-phrase your limiting beliefs. Re-write them in a way that serves you best. What do you choose to believe instead? How can you rephrase these to motivate yourself?

Go ahead. Turn the negative above into positive below:

1.

_____

2.

_____

3.

_____

4.

_____

5.

_____

Once you have written your responses, repeat them as often as you can, like a mantra, until they become a part of you. These new beliefs are to be carried with your well-formed outcome. There are only five here. You will want to pay attention to your thoughts, and soon, you will be amazed at how easy it is to turn a limiting belief into a positive statement that serves you.

You will become a Professional Beliefs Transformer. Watch your life go from a negative to a positive trend.

KEY CONCEPTS:

NEGATIVE TO POSITIVE

Your lack of success may have led you to create some limiting beliefs regarding clean living.

These beliefs dictate the way you act. You need to change them to support your desires as opposed to standing in the way of realizing your goals.

You can start changing a belief by linguistically re-phrasing it.

PART 7

THE "A"

CHAPTER 32:

ACTUALIZE

"Affirm it, visualize it, believe and it will actualize itself."

- Norman Vincent Peale

The third component of the D.N.A. System is ACTUALIZE. Now that you have cleaned out your negative emotions and limiting beliefs, you will learn how to install the new desires you uncovered in the first section. Various techniques will guide you into programming the NEW YOU.

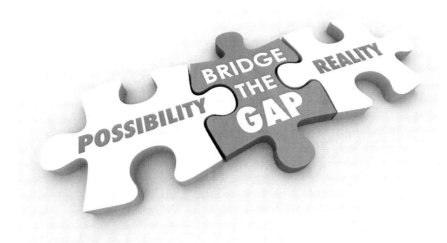

The ACTUALIZE section will help you to re-define the choices you will continue to make once your new desires are installed. This section will also prepare you for alternative options in the event you face unexpected situations. You will learn how to become accountable to yourself and feel authentic by feeding your brain daily with positive thoughts.

You have already generated your DESIRES and created a NEW YOU. You are now ready to install your desires and program your brain with what you want. This section will teach you how to implement and cement your desires. You have chosen your new kitchen. You know exactly what you want. You removed the old cupboards, and now it is time to install the new ones and lay down the marble countertop.

This section will allow you to build a strong new foundation for clean living. You will also have tools to become your best and ensure that the emotions of failure don't return. You will develop resilience which will enable you to deflect negative energy and remain positive.

KEY CONCEPTS

ACTUALIZE

The third component of the D.N.A. System is the ACTUALIZE part. You will learn in this section how to implement and program your desires into your brain.

"You have your identity when you find out, not what you can keep your mind on, but what you can't keep your mind off."

- A.R. Ammons

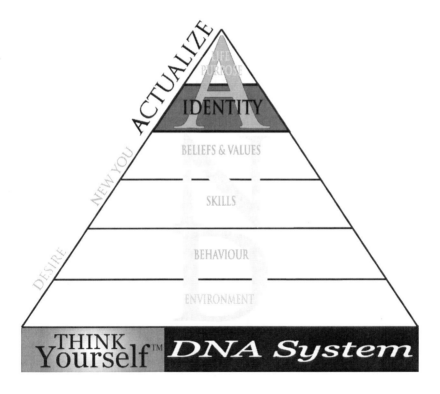

The next neurological level is Identity. At this level, we integrate all previous neurological levels. The knowledge you have accumulated from the four previous levels is contributing to creating who you are now. YOU.

You are becoming more aligned with your true self, and your life reflects that alignment. Your behaviours are now in line with your beliefs and values, which allows you to use your skills in an environment that supports your identity. You are the result of these levels combined. What you manifest externally represents your most authentic desires. Life becomes more joyful, playful and relaxed.

In this section, we will help you determine your identity. The following section will help clarify and anchor your new identity.

Who am I?

> *Example:*

> *I am a mother and I lead my children by example, living a clean life. I am an inspiration to them so that they, in turn, will also embrace clean living.*

What do I love about who I am?

> *Example:*

> *I love how I allow myself to be a student. I am willing to taste new food and try new recipes that will nourish me, and ultimately how I feel.*

Is there a portion of who I am that I do not like? Is part of 'me' missing, lost, or as of yet unexplored?

Example:

I would rather have more will power.

I have always wanted to run a half-marathon.

"Who am I to be Brilliant? Gorgeous?
Talented? The Real question is: Who am I
NOT to be?"

- Marianne Williamson

When do you feel that your environment, behaviours, skills, beliefs and values are aligned?

Example:

When I prepare a healthy recipe with confidence and my family loves it, I feel that my identity is rewarded.

When I do something that I am good at, in an environment that supports what is important to me, I feel that my identity is integrated.

When do you feel that two parts of your identity are colliding?

Example:

When we are running out of time, I find myself stopping at the drive-thru to feed my kids on the way to the soccer practice and it goes against my desire to keep my family healthy.

Which of my identities do I want to be more of, or can I merge both identities so that I don't have to choose?

Example:

As a busy parent, there are times where I am going to be under pressure to prepare a clean meal for my family. I am willing to learn what clean, ready-prepared food options there are at a healthy grocery store, so I can still offer something healthy.

KEY CONCEPTS

IDENTITY

The answers to these questions will allow you to combine everything you have learned so far to find your own identity.

The integration of all parts of yourself allows you to start embracing each part fully and live true to your complete identity.

CHAPTER 34:

SELF-CARE

*"The most powerful relationship you will ever
have is the relationship with yourself."*

- Diane Von Furstenberg

Now that you are clear about you who are, we are introducing you to an easy technique to protect and preserve your newly found identity. To have the vitality needed to ACTUALIZE your positive outcome, you need to commit first and foremost to your own self-care.

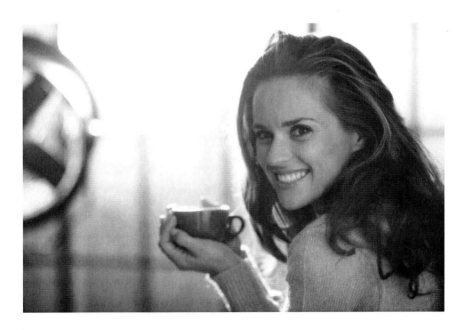

Self-care is nourishment, and proper nourishment leads to a state of thriving. It is therefore imperative that you be mindful of the influences you allow into your life. You will agree by now that this book is indeed more about the mind than it is about the body. However, a healthy body is imperative and inherent to any goal. Which immensely wealthy, successful... and sick person would not give all their fortune to get their health back?

Commitment to self-care equals a commitment to your own identity.

Here are several practical strategies you can use for self-care.

FOOD

There is no debate that food has the power to heal or hurt you. Since you are trying to embrace a clean lifestyle, to bring yourself to optimal wellness, here are several practical strategies to help you understand the power of food:

- Source your food well, so you know where it comes from and how it was produced.

- Eat whole food, transformed as little as possible and strive to eat mostly plant-based foods.

- Drink more water. Ideally about 3 liters per day.

- Focus on leafy and green vegetables as well as coloured fruits and vegetables for maximum nutrition.

- Be mindful of what is on your plate and how much. Half your plate should be vegetables, a quarter should be protein and the last quarter can be a starch.

- Minimize consumption of refined foods, including flour and sugar

- Stay away from packaged foods, particularly those with ingredients you can't spell or pronounce.

- Include healthy fats to help you maintain a lean, healthy body.

- Limit alcohol consumption.

- Know yourself and understand that each food behaves differently in each of you.

These are just a few suggestions about food. For more, refer to Tosca's nutrition and recipe books that can be found at www. toscareno.com or *THINK Yourself*® *HEALTHY* that can be found at www.thinkyourself.com.

MOVEMENT

Choose a way to move your body. You may like to run, participate in spin or yoga class, or go for a walk. Just move in ways that make you feel vital (yes, sex counts! – Stay tuned for *THINK Yourself*® *SEXY* coming up in the THINK Yourself® series).

Movement sends fresh new energy to the brain so that it can process and retain information faster and better. Therefore, you will experience optimal gains from this book if you intentionally move your body either before, or after, tackling sections of this book. It will enhance your experience, clear out the cobwebs, and help to create a clean slate.

DAILY GRATITUDE

There are many benefits to creating the habit of journaling daily. Respond to these questions at the end of each day. You can also choose to get *THINK Yourself® GRATEFUL*, the daily journal from the THINK Yourself® series.

MY "HAVE-DONE-LIST" FOR TODAY

I accomplished this today:

_____

I took this step towards my goal:

_____

MY "HAVE-BEEN-LIST" FOR TODAY

Here is a positive emotion I chose to feel today:

_____

Here is a new positive belief I chose to create today or existing positive belief that served me today:

_____

MY GRATITUDES FOR TODAY

Today, I am Grateful for:

_____

MY PLAN FOR TOMORROW

Tomorrow, I will end the day having done this important thing:

_____

SLEEP

Sleep when you need it. It is not the quantity of sleep; it is the quality of it. Nothing will bolster your creativity, immune system and productivity more. The body knows what it needs to function optimally. Let your body decide when it is time to get up, not your alarm clock. We are not saying that you should sleep in until 11am or noon every day. We know you have to get up and go to work and accomplish the million things you need to on a daily basis. What we want to address here are two important notions about sleep.

The first one, is to observe and track your sleep. Notice how you feel after seven hours of sleep, eight hours of sleep, nine hours of sleep. Soon, you will know your optimal number of hours, in order to feel energized when you get up, and maintain your activity level in order to have a productive day. When you have identified the number of hours of sleep you need, just count back to know what time you need to be in bed the night before. For example, if you need to get up at six a.m. and you need seven hours of sleep, that means that you need to plan to be in bed by eleven p.m.

The second thing we want to address is the quality of your sleep. You may say: "Well, it is not because I am in bed at 11 p.m. that I am *asleep* at 11 p.m. I also may get up a few times during the night so my total number of hours asleep may not be seven hours." Pay attention to the thoughts that keep you from falling asleep and start delegating some of your *thinking* to your unconscious mind. You can avoid time wasted trying to fall asleep by using your personal assistant. Just place an order every night as soon as you lay your head on the pillow. Say to yourself: "While I fall into a deep and comfortable sleep in a few minutes, I would like you to do all my thinking and have some answers for me when I wake up refreshed tomorrow morning. I will sleep through the night and get a full night of rejuvenating sleep." This will make sure you trust your unconscious mind to deliver in the morning and let you get a full restful sleep. Your personal assistant and your chef know the answers to your questions and know everything about your schedule and your to-do list. Let them do the work while you recharge.

SAY YES

Say YES to new opportunities, things that scare you, situations that support you and anything that makes you curious. You will then be better able to create a clean life, *by design*, not by default.

SAY NO

Say NO to those people and situations that no longer serve you. Recognize when you need to pull back to take care of yourself. Say no to things that stand in the way of having space and energy to focus on the things you want.

"If it is not a Hell Yes! Then it is a no." –
Nathalie Plamondon-Thomas

ASK AND RECEIVE

Asking for and receiving what you need is a mark of social acuity. 'Asking and Receiving' may be a hurdle for you, because you are biologically programmed to give and often don't feel worthy to receive. Women, especially, are often identified as 'the nurturer'. You cannot be successful if you do not first practice asking and receiving. It begins by being mindful of the multiple opportunities that present themselves for you to learn how to ask for what you need. When you receive what you asked for, receive your abundance with grace.

USE THE D.N.A. SYSTEM

Use the tools of this book! There are multiple layers that can be applied to every area of your life. When you focus the tools of this book in one area of your life, they will influence your way of thinking, feeling and seeing yourself and the world around you. That can only impact other areas of your life in a positive way until you can intentionally refocus your efforts in the next area of your life! You can apply everything you have learned in this book to your love life, your career, your relation with your family, your wealth and living a clean life.

KEY CONCEPTS:

SELF-CARE

Proper nutrition, movement, daily gratitude, sleep, saying yes and saying no, asking, receiving and using the tools in this book will help you to live an optimal life.

CHAPTER 35:

LIFE PURPOSE

*"Here is the test to find whether your mission on
earth is finished. If you're alive, it isn't."*

- Richard Bach

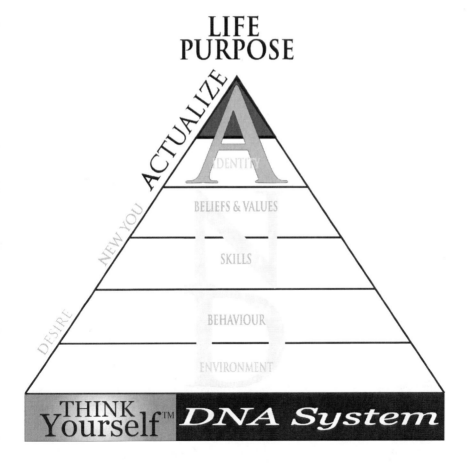

The last level of the pyramid is Life Purpose. Finding your identity is the ultimate condition for you to experience happiness. You need to be able to be yourself and to love yourself. The remaining layer, once you are living your full identity, is to turn towards the world and find your purpose. Who else are you serving? Whom do you inspire?

KNOWING YOUR PURPOSE
KEEPS YOU GOING

Imagine for a moment that you are driving home after work and there is a tree blocking the road. You can't get to your house. Are you going to turn around and say: "Oh no, I will never be able to go home again! That's too bad because I really loved my kids and my spouse. I will miss them. Now I have to find a new home and buy all new furniture to fill it."

This is not how it would unfold? You would either turn around and find an alternate route, park the car and walk home or find a chainsaw to cut the tree and get to your home. When the stakes are high, you always find a way. No tree could get you to abandon your family and home. You want to make your desire for a clean life just as compelling as going back home so that no obstacle can make you decide to give up.

LEAD WITH YOUR 'WHY'

Now that you have answered several fundamental questions about your environment, behaviours, skills, beliefs and values, you have opened your mind, and discovered your identity. You now have access to most pieces of the puzzle. Nathalie's friend Kelly does puzzles all the time. Kelly has a process for making puzzles. She starts by looking at the picture on the cover and noticing the big picture ahead of time. She observes the edges, top and bottom, other details and each area of the final image. Then she starts taking pieces out of the box. First, she picks only the pieces with flat edges that will ultimately the frame. Once the frame has been built, she takes more pieces out and selects those with similar colours and puts them together. Each step of her puzzle making process gets her closer to the final picture.

Answering the questions in this book is similar to Kelly's puzzle making process. Answering the questions, taking the steps and building the layers that are being installed in your brain brings you closer to your goal. The complete picture is starting to come together as a result. You have created the frame, filled in most of the picture, and now you are down to the last few pieces that will make the image bright and brilliant.

Michelangelo believed that in every chunk of raw marble, the final image already existed. His only task was to reveal it. The same is true of you. You have your "art" inside of you. The reason you are doing what you do lives at the heart of you. Your life purpose drives you forward. Your answers are already inside you somewhere at the "bottom of a messy drawer" but there was so much clutter accumulated in the drawer that you could no longer see the clearly.

Answering a WHY question might have been challenging for you at the beginning of this book. Now that you have all the pieces of the puzzle, you know what you want and what is important to you. You have cleared limiting beliefs and negative emotions, out and you know who you are. Answers to your many questions now start to come naturally.

You now must locate and extract from the box the main pieces of the puzzle that represent your 'why'. The next series of questions will further open up your unconscious mind to move you closer to optimal wellness.

Why do you want the things you want?

Example:

I want the things I want because my desire is to watch my daughters grow up and have children of their own. I want to fully participate in every minute of life.

What do you love?

Example:

I love being a role model for friends and family and make it seem possible for others.

Nathalie's answer:

I love loving people because I want to love them. I love the love that I give more than the love I receive.

Tosca's answer:

I love the reward of loving someone, even a stranger because when we love, we close the space between us, becoming stronger, like the pieces of a completed puzzle.

Who do you love?

Example:

I love my children and family. I love people who know me from the inside out and like me anyway.

Nathalie's answer:

I love my husband, family and friends and those around me who welcome my message, even if I don't have a personal connection with every one of my followers.

Tosca's answer:

I love those I serve, including my children, family, friends, audience and complete strangers. I love people who help grow my mind, even if I don't know them personally.

What brings you joy? A sense of Purpose? Peace?

Example:

My children. Helping others. Creating something new. Acknowledging someone else's goodness. Knowing how to heal my body and my mind.

What do you know for sure? And what is your 'Big Why'?

Example:

I know for sure ... that I have a perspective on life and gifts to offer that no one else on this planet has in quite the same way. I know that I am unique, which in no way diminishes the person next to me. They are also unique.

My BIG WHY is to create the legacy of a better world for my children, where they can more easily live their own gifts, and find joy in helping others.

Life purpose is all about what is beyond you. It is an extension of you that serves someone other than yourself. Beyond your identity, who else are you serving?

How are you a contributor?

Example:

I contribute by living my true life-purpose which helps those around me and gives other people permission to do the same.

Now that you have tapped into all six layers of your brain, let's go back to chapter 27 where you wrote your positive outcome. Having explored the levels of your brain, you now can expand on your outcome. Use the following exercise to give more substance to your goal.

Exercise:

Project yourself into the future. Imagine you have achieved your goal. What does your environment look like? What are you doing? What skills do you have? What do you believe? Who are you? Who are you serving?

Re-write your positive outcome:

Example:

I get up in the morning feeling rested after a long night's sleep and I am excited about my day. I feel I am using my skills and what I am good at in my tasks and have set up an environment filled with positive people. I also have the resources I need. I feel that my clean habits fit with my values and what is important to me. I feel good about myself. I have abundant energy and live a clean life. My skin glows. I am experiencing a life altering shift and feel at ease and comfortable with my life. Moreover, I feel that I contribute to the world in a meaningful way because I am achieving my life purpose. I am my very best self.

You will now continue your journey in the ACTUALIZE section and complete the D.N.A. System using tools, techniques and success strategies. This practice will fully immerse you in your new-found identity and drive you to live your life's purpose. Acquiring the knowledge is one thing. Now we will teach you how to maintain it and ACTUALIZE it in your life.

KEY CONCEPTS:

LIFE PURPOSE

Finding your life's purpose allows you to step into the highest expression of yourself.

Living your purpose is to step into your Leader shoes and ask yourself: "Who else am I serving?"

Beyond being your own personal best, beyond your identity, to whom or what do you contribute?

CHAPTER 36:

CHANGING OUR EATING PATTERNS TO HELP HEAL THE PLANET

"The Greatest Threat to Our Planet Is the Belief That Someone Else Will Save It"

- Robert Swan

Today our planet faces an extreme condition the likes of which has never been witnessed before. Global Warming is a phrase uppermost in everyone's mind. The stakes are high. Global Warming is happening so fast that sea levels are rising, and the impacts of climate change are more significant than initially imagined. There are fears that we are close to "the end" if we don't quickly make drastic changes.

An enterprising Californian, Paul Hawken, is an American environmentalist, entrepreneur, activist and author of the New York Times bestselling book *Drawdown*. He recently took matters into his own hands, so great was his concern over our Earth. In this game-changing book – and yes we are getting to the point of food – Hawken makes over 100 recommendations to curb the emission of greenhouse gases, using scientific models.

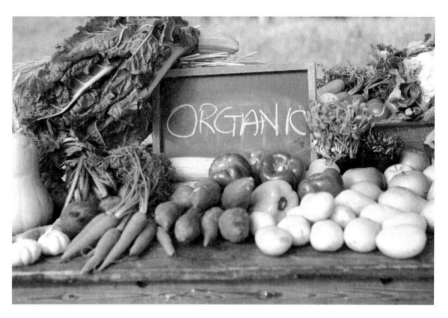

His goal is "drawdown." Drawdown is the point in time at which greenhouse gases peak and begin to decline on a year-to-year basis. Why this matters to the readers of this book is that the main contributing factors to Global Warming are food related. This means that while food is among the greatest contributing factors to the environmental shifts in our planet, we can also change them. They include, in ranked order, from creating the most significant impact to less so:

SOLUTION	RANKING	GIGATONS REDUCED
Refrigeration	1	89.74
Wind turbines	2	84.60
Reduced food waste	3	70.53
Plant-rich diet	4	66.11
Tropical forests	5	61.23
Educating girls	6	59.60
Family planning	7	36.90
Solar farms	8	31.19
Silvopasture	10	24.60

It is clear that among the top solutions to reducing greenhouse gases, 4 of the 10 activities involve making changes to how the population handles, grows and processes food. This means that with renewed practices in these areas Drawdown can be reduced by as much as 287.61 Gigatons (adding refrigeration + reduced food waste + plant-rich diet + tropical forests).

Looking at the Global Warming situation as one gigantic problem doesn't offer much hope. It feels overwhelming and impossible to contribute in a significant way. However, when you break it down (as you do when you are making neurological behavioural changes to your brain) what each of you can do to help solve the problem, is substantial given that there are seven billion of you on the planet. When you commit to wasting less food, properly disposing of old refrigerators and consuming more plant-based food, rather than animal-based, it is easy to see how much power each of you has in your hands. The cumulative effect is enormous.

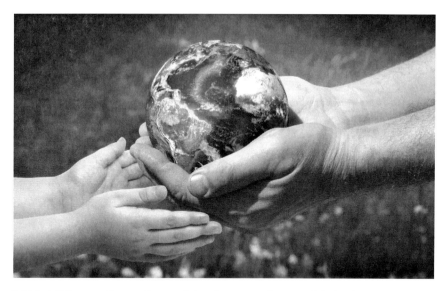

With billions of people on this planet eating multiple times per day, the opportunity to positively affect the planet is immense. According to the World Health Organization, only 10 – 15% of daily calories need to come from protein. While it is true that no civilization since the dawn of time has thrived without animal-based protein, a well-planned plant-based diet can readily support protein needs. A World Resources Institute report found that "ambitious animal protein reduction" focused on reducing overconsumption of animal-based foods … holds great promise for ensuring a sustainable future for global food supply and the planet."

You don't need to wait for a big organization with a fancy plan to tell you what to do. You can begin to draw down on greenhouse gas emissions right now. Buy only enough food to get you through a few days, much like the practice in Europe. In Tosca's native Holland, refrigerators are about half the size of refrigerators sold here. Consumers only buy enough food for a few days thereby reducing food waste. Regular market days are a feature of Dutch life so fresh produce is always available. This is a common practice in numerous other countries. Buying fresh produce and goods helps to keep food from landing in landfills.

Adopting a plant-rich diet ranks 4th on the list of Drawdown solutions. This is surprisingly easy to do. Many have already adopted a Meatless Monday into their weekly menu plans. Including a meatless or vegetarian option, every other day can significantly reduce pressure on this fragile planet. There are many vegetarian platforms and resources to access easy recipes and alternative to meat.

In Tosca's household, she has a practice of eating every meal until dinnertime as a vegetarian. Then 60 % of all her dinners in the week are meat free. She has written a Vegetarian Cookbook to support her beliefs, and she wishes to do as much for the planet as possible. This includes growing her own vegetables in her garden and composting all kitchen waste. There are no pesticides or toxins in her little plot. Nathalie doesn't eat meat. All her meals are vegetarian. Her first rule is: "No animal needs to die for me to eat." She considers the planet and her health when making food choices. When she has company, she sources organic meat or impresses her guests with a squash and quinoa dish and a few of her delicious salads. Taking care of the planet begins in Tosca's and Nathalie's kitchen. And yours.

Eating Clean® is Eating Green. In Tosca's dinner plate formula, she places a heavy emphasis on eating greens as follows.

30% fat + 30% protein + 40% carbohydrate
(20% greens + 20% grains and dairy) =
Body Beautiful Body Healthy

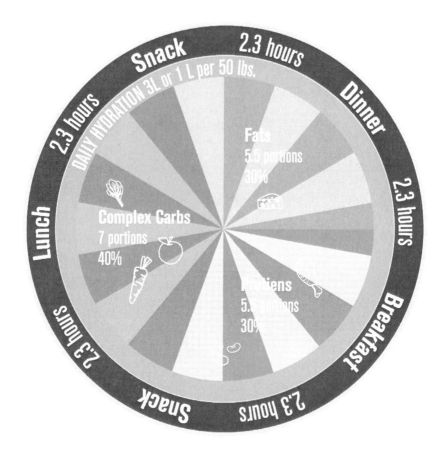

Artwork by Kelsey-Lynn Coradetti

It is Tosca's deeply seated belief that you must consume more green plant matter.

Elizabeth Kolbert, an environmental writer for the *New Yorker*, recently wrote: a "… matter-of-fact accounting of how little humans are willing to change to protect species other than their own." Her book, *The Sixth Extinction*, compels Tosca to do better, to preserve not only plants and animals but ourselves. Kolbert makes Tosca want to take up the fight to preserve something living, green, viable and beautiful, even if only in her half-acre patch of dirt. You and I must have some sense of control, of stepping up to serve up a message worth leaving to our children and theirs.

KEY CONCEPTS:

Clean living includes caring for your environment.

Global warming is an imminent threat.

Among the top solutions to reducing greenhouse gases, food ranks as a top priority

Eating organic food, efficient refrigeration, reduced food waste, plant-rich diet and tropical forests contribute, not only to your health, but to the planet's preservation.

CHAPTER 37:

ACT & MERGE

"Acting like someone you're not is exactly what it takes to realize you're capable of more than you ever knew."

- Rob Sheridan

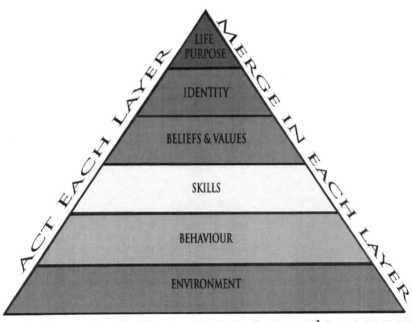

LAYERS OF A PERSON'S SELF

Action is imperative to actualizing your New You. It is not enough to read and reflect. Real and lasting change require that you move outside of your comfort zone and take the initial steps to realizing the new you. An action is a tool to do exactly that! Sometimes you get stuck in "analysis paralysis", or a relationship with perfectionism that leads to procrastination. To actualize, you need to stop thinking and start doing.

273

Through the D.NA. System, you have learned that your Self is built with different layers. This next exercise will place you in each neurological level for you to break down every layer of yourself and assign a new reality to each part of you. You will assume a new environment, new behaviours, skills, beliefs and values.

You will use the six neurological levels of the D.N.A. System to take action and figure out what you need to achieve your vision.

Consider the following example. Some countries have analyzed and tried to copy Michael Phelps' record breaking swimming techniques. Experts considered his environment. They wanted to know everything about it from the type of water Phelps swam in to the temperature of that water. What was his swimsuit made of? What foods did he eat? What was the volume of calories he consumed every day? Then they looked at his behaviours. The studied how Phelps performed each stroke from the minutest details like at what exact moment did his hand enter the water to which finger touched first? They studied how Phelps stood just before diving into the water? Taking their observations of Phelps behaviours they copied his skills. In what did Phelps excel? Is it when he makes his flip turns? When in the race did Phelps get the lead? Is it in the first half or the second half? What did he do exceptionally well that differentiates him from his competition so much that no one has been able to outperform his numerous record-breaking swims?

The "spying" techniques of these curious countries stopped at this point. Officials did not go beyond the first three layers of the brain. They did not know what Michael Phelps has INSIDE his head. What does Phelps think when he trains? What is important to him? What does he value? What does he believe? What is in his head just before a race? You can readily imagine that all Phelps must see is himself executing a winning race every time. He probably already sees himself on the podium with the gold medal around his neck. What is his identity? When he responds to the question: "Who am I?" He must respond: "I am the fastest swimmer in the world." And what is his life purpose? Who else is he serving? Does he inspire young athletes? Is he doing this for his son that he is now teaching to swim? We must ask these questions to be able to get to each layer of the mind and install a new excellent serving habit.

Nathalie often asks questions of her clients, and for many, they simply don't have answers. Then she asks: "If you knew, what would that be?" Sometimes, this question works, sometimes, there is still no answer. Then she asks: " What advice would you give someone in your situation?" The thought of being able to help someone they care about is often enough to generate a response. That is true for the majority of the population. However, occasionally there is no answer.

Nathalie then asks the magic questions: "Do you know someone who has been successful at this and what would they do in your situation?" All of a sudden, the responses are flowing. They say: "Well, they would certainly do such and such, they would tell me to do this and that, etc." It is amusing how, once they put themselves in someone else's shoes, they have all the answers. They know exactly what someone else would do. Yet, the other person did not tell them what they did or have done or would do. The answers were inside the client's head all along. They did not think they had them. You too, have everything you need inside. Go ahead. Ask yourself the questions.

What is the environment of people living a clean life? Where are they? Who is with them? Where do they hang out?

Example:

They must be surrounded with like-minded people seeking wellness.

Their kitchen is filled with nutritious food.

Their environment, supports their clean living.

There are no pizza boxes, packaged food, soda, or other junk foods in their home.

They hang out at the gym and outdoors.

What are the behaviours of clean living people? What do they do? What are their actions?

Examples:

They are planning their meals.

They seek out and learn about new foods and healthy ingredient.

They exercise on a regular basis.

They source their food wisely and even grow their own.

What are the skills of clean living people? What are they good at?

Examples:

They don't arrive at meal times and try to figure out what they will eat on the fly. They are not leaving it to chance.

They are not at the mercy of a vending machine or a drive-thru.

They are actively planning and consciously selecting everything that will nourish them.

They are disciplined.

They are skilled at creating recipes.

The sum total of their choices supports an active lifestyle.

They make a priority of moving daily thinking it is a privilege not a punishment.

What are the beliefs and values of clean living people? What do they believe? What is important to them?

Example:

They believe in themselves.

They believe they can do anything.

Their health is important to them.

They believe that it is possible for them to live a clean life.

They believe they can constantly learn about wellness.

They take responsibility for their self-care themselves, they don't believe that it is the responsibility of the health care system to make them well.

They don't believe that being sick is normal. It isn't.

They believe that food is their primary medicine.

Who are they? When they say: ''I am...'' fill in the blank.

Example:

I am healthy.

I am confident.

I am curious about learning more.

I am organized.

I am fit.

I am free.

I am the evidence of my healthy choices.

I am strong.

I am alive.

I am awesome.

I am energetic.

I am the best expression of myself.

I am in love with who I see in the mirror.

What is their life purpose? Who else are they serving?

Example:

They inspire others to live to their fullest potential.

They inspire their children and family members.

They are serving humanity by taking the burden off of the health care system.

They are contributing to the survival of our planet.

They are raising the bar on what is possible for wellness in general.

ACT

Now that you have a few answers on paper, you can try it out for yourself. As you know by now, your unconscious mind can process so much more information than what you can write down. Immerse yourself in each of these neurological levels to adopt them as your own.

Start to adopt these behaviours in their environment, acquiring the necessary skills and beliefs so that you can identify yourself as a clean living individual and start serving and inspiring those around you.

If closing your eyes and doing the mental work on your own seems difficult or too abstract, you can get support by downloading the THINK Yourself® CLEAN video series on www.thinkyourself.com to have access to Nathalie and Tosca's videos to guide you through the exercises and processes of this book.

KEY CONCEPTS:

ACT & MERGE - PROGRAM YOUR BRAIN

To fully integrate your desired outcome, you must act as if you have already achieved your goals and immerse yourself in each neurological level to embody each area of yourself. This process allows you to transform your actions into a fully merged reality.

CHAPTER 38:
ANTICIPATE

"Success in life is not how well we execute plan A;
it's how smoothly we cope with plan B."

- Sarah Ban Breathnach

Anticipate. There is a good chance the reason you haven't been living clean in the past is that you were unaware there were other choices and other alternatives to the behaviours that were causing you to fail. You had beliefs that were not serving you and part of your identity was yet uncovered. You may not have had a clear understanding of your Why. This strong sense of purpose will give you the energy you need when you face an obstacle.

It is not your personal history that makes you who you are. It is your response to it with the choices that you have available at the time. You can choose what behaviour you want to execute and program them in advance. What are the obstacles that you can anticipate will be in your way?

You have the mental skills to know what you don't want and to replace that with what you do want. The following exercise will allow you to be in charge of the change that will happen to you, the direction you will go, and what you will become.

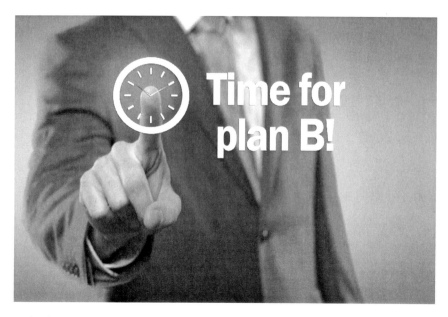

It is time to foresee what can stand between you and your desired outcome. Do you remember the tree on the road as you were on your way home? What will stand between you and your goal of living a clean life? In this chapter, you will develop a Plan B.

HERE ARE SOME EXAMPLES:

Imagine you had intended to do meal prepping this weekend, but your friends showed up with a wine bottle. Now what? It is decision-making time. Are you going to join them? Are you going to have one glass? Are you going to suggest that you all hang out for a long visit in the kitchen while you do your meal prep? Are you going to use this as an opportunity to introduce them to clean foods?

If you noticed that you were "weak" (making poor choices) while choosing what to eat from a buffet at a function, you will now always eat before you go and avoid showing up starving.

If your downfall has been the fact that you tend to go off track frequently, you will now know to always carry healthy food with you to avoid eating junk food.

If you work in an office where a lady comes to your floor every day at 2 pm with a tray of coffee and doughnuts, plan to visit the bathroom, or go anywhere far away from the temptation, at this specific time.

Have a "What If" plan. What if you get called into a meeting at the pub at lunchtime when you were planning to eat your healthy homemade lunch? Your Plan B will be to order the soup or a small healthy appetizer and eat your lunch later on in the afternoon.

What if everyone is going out for brunch on Saturday morning when you had planned to do a workout? You will take an hour to exercise and then meet them later, as people always arrive late anyway. By the time they order, you will get there just in time for the food or better yet, eat at home quickly before you go. What you want really is to hang out with your friends, not the food.

Always take control and have a backup plan. Don't let yourself be surprised. You know what distractions are presented to you! Prepare, prepare, prepare. You should not be surprised that you need to eat at least three times a day. You have pretty much been operating with the same body all our lives. Noon hour shouldn't come with a sense of being caught off guard that it is now lunchtime. Always know what you will eat.

List some obstructions that could get in the way of your CLEAN LIVING.

OBSTRUCTIONS

Anticipate the things that could get in the way

1. _____

2. _____

3. _____

4. _____

5. _____

Find an alternative for them – what's your Plan B?

1. _____

2. _____

3. _____

4. _____

5. _____

This tool will help you plan for new, better serving behaviours. Now we know we can plan ahead for behaviours. But can we also prepare for our emotions?

KEY CONCEPTS

ANTICIPATE

You probably know some scenarios that could get in the way of your new lifestyle.

By anticipating these situations, you can plan ahead what you will choose to do, instead of falling back on your old negative behaviour.

CHAPTER 39:

ANCHORING

*"Courage is like a muscle. We strengthen it
with use."*

- Ruth Gordon

Here is an exercise to trigger a positive feeling with the process of anchoring. You can use it whenever you are about to make a choice related to your clean living journey. An emotional feeling can trigger a physical response, and the reverse can also happen. A physical stimulus can trigger an emotional state.

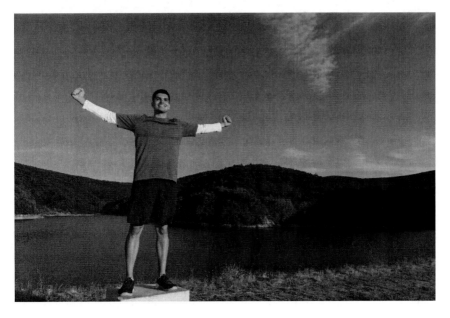

Step One:
Recall the positive feeling to be anchored

Imagine a movie screen in front of you with a control button connected to what you see on the screen. Go back in your mind to a time, a specific time, when you had a wonderful experience. Feel the feelings that you felt back then. Perhaps you will remember a scene when you were on a roll with your exercise routine and getting results. Or a memory of a time you were successful at meal prepping or a time you know that you had lots of willpower.

Step Two:
Amplify the positive feeling to be anchored

Picture the image getting bigger and closer. Live it as the feeling increases. Be "associated", that is, be the main character, seeing the experience through your own eyes - as opposed to being a third person looking at yourself, "dissociated". As this happens, imagine that the control button says 'awesome' and slowly imagine turning it up. To make it feel even more real, as the feeling intensifies, make the physical gesture with the button with your hand. As you turn it up, at the rate that suits the changes, allow that exhilarating memory to get closer, bigger and brighter. Add colour to it. Make it shine. Notice the details. Hear a voice in your head saying: "I am awesome! I feel amazing!"

Step Three:
Anchor

At this moment, when you are thoroughly imprinted with the feeling, apply pressure to a part of your body, which will become the kinesthetic anchor for this remarkable state of mind. You can choose the anchor to be a specific spot on your hand, on your knuckle, on the back of your neck, etc. Choose a particular spot that you can recall quickly. Avoid common anchors like pressing your hands together, which you usually do in other states (i.e. when you are nervous or when you are cold) because that could send wrong messages to your brain without you noticing. Choose something specific that will only be used to recall positive feelings.

Step Four:
Neutral

Enjoy this sensation for an instant, then release the anchor and let your body come back to a neutral state.

Step Five:
Repeat

Repeat the process a few times. It is important to apply the anchor at the peak of the emotional state. It is essential that you repeat the process at least three times to avoid sending mixed messages to your brain. Before moving on to step five, you must make sure that your brain knows exactly what to do when you press the anchor.

Step Six:
Test

To verify that the anchoring was successful, remember a moment when you were not at your best. Go there in your mind and feel how it felt. In this negative state, the application of pressure on the anchor will reverse your state and make you feel wonderful instead. Press the anchor as you say to yourself: "I am awesome! I feel amazing" You will find yourself feeling as ecstatic as before.

You can choose anywhere on your body as an anchor point. Nathalie uses a physical anchor on herself. She has a spot right behind her neck that she presses firmly with three fingers every time she is in a fantastic mood including: when she finishes a conference or a seminar that went well, witnessing a client succeeding in something, at the end of a great fitness class where she was at her best, when something significant happens to her or simply when she feels like a million bucks! She has been anchoring these feelings right behind her neck for years. And now, whenever she needs a boost, whenever some external pressure comes to her, whenever there is a tree on the road, she presses the back of her neck with her three fingers and her brain thinks that it needs to generate these exhilarating feelings, which works every time. She immediately gets a rush of beautiful warm sensations, which helps her go through whatever is presenting itself to her at the time.

Remember to keep adding on to your anchor, anytime you experience a wonderful feeling. First, amplify it and then anchor it. Keep stacking more and more so that you make your anchor robust and powerful.

SPACIAL ANCHORING

You have just learned a technique called physical anchoring. You can also use a space anchor. Here is the process that we call the Clean Circle.

Step One:
Set up the space

Imagine a circle big enough so that you could easily step into it. Give it a colour and visualize it. Place it on the floor in front of you and stand just behind it.

Step Two:
Recall the positive feeling to be anchored.

Think of a specific time when you were at your best or when you were easily able to perform the behaviour that you are trying to achieve. For example, if you are feeling lazy and don't feel like exercising, think of a time where you were exercising regularly and effortlessly. You can also imagine the outcome if you cannot find a memory of it. Make a compelling movie in your head of how you want to feel. Get into that specific feeling, the same way as above, being associated in the memory, seeing it through your own eyes and increasing the awesomeness of the event.

Step Three:
Anchor

When you are at the peak of the moment, physically step into the Clean Circle that you previously placed on the floor in front of you. Power pose by standing tall, rolling your shoulders back and keeping your head up. Hold the feeling there for a moment until you feel that it starts fading away. When it does, leave the feeling in the circle as you step out. Repeat a few times to anchor the feeling in the circle.

Step Four:
Test

Get into a neutral feeling. Step into the Clean Circle. Notice if your mood changes and adopts the feelings that were left for you in your circle. Whenever you feel that you need extra willpower, take out your imaginary Clean Circle and step into it.

You can use the same process for many situations and you may also have different coloured circles to match various desired states.

KEY CONCEPTS:

ANCHORING

You can store positive feelings in a physical or spatial anchor and recall them when you need them simply by triggering the anchor.

The anchor can be a physical point on your body or the action of stepping into an imaginary circle on the floor.

CHAPTER 40:

ONGOING PROCESS

"In the marathon of life, there is no finish line."

- Bill Courtney

Are you fixed for good now? You just programmed your brain so that must be the end, right? You are good to go forever, no? In the same way you cannot eat your next twenty-one meals for the whole week today and not have to eat again this week, you will need to feed your mind again on a daily basis. Fifty percent of people who begin a self-directed program will drop out in the first 6 months. When you are not being monitored, you decrease your chances of success, because you lack the mental key.

Is reading this book enough? Can you store it on a shelf now and completely forget about it? This would then become 'shelf-help'. Is answering the questions and doing any of these processes once enough? You must keep re-doing them until they are part of your way of being, until they become your daily routine. Do them until you have a natural habit of amplifying and anchoring positive feelings. Do them until you can easily perform a successful behaviour and make it become yours.

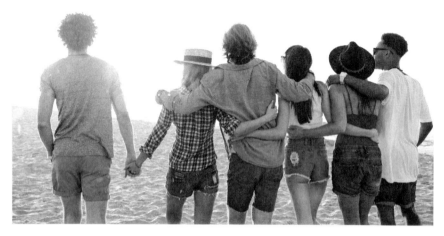

Keep surrounding yourself with people seeking wellness just as you are. In the same way, you need to eat healthy food every day; you also need to feed your brain every day.

Now that you are aware of the art of programming your brain and are excited and motivated to try it for yourself, you may wonder how to keep the positive energy going. Often, despite our best intentions, life can get in the way. How do you master programming your brain?

Nathalie and Tosca have developed the habit of continuing to feed their souls with books, podcasts, audiobooks and they attend seminars and conferences. Jack Canfield once said: "You can't put your hand in a bucket of glue, without some of that glue sticking to your hand." Hanging out with successful people and reading their biographies, their stories of how they did it and what lessons they learned needs to be part of your strategy.

Here are some of the authors' favourite books:

- *Change your Brain, Change your Body* by Daniel G. Amen

- *How to Create the Life you Want* by Wayne Dwyer

- *How to Overcome your Self Limiting Beliefs & Achieve Any thing You Want* by Omar Johnson

- *Mindset* by Carol S. Dweck

- *The Art of Thinking Clearly* by Rolf Dobelli

- *Sugar Blues* by William Dufty

- *Whole Food* by Paul Pitchford

- *Power vs Force* by David Hawkins

- *Whole* by Colin Campbell

- *Nourishing Traditions* by Sally Fallon

- *You can Heal your Life* by Louise Hay

Start your day off by listening to positive, motivating audiobooks or Podcasts. Hire a coach. Or join a class with a group of friends who will help you stay on track and motivated.

What are you going to do to stay motivated? It's easy after you've just been fed positive information and tools. Your homework now is to put into action the tools you will need to stay motivated. Getting into a good state is mandatory when we are learning and implementing new positive habits.

What are you going to do to stay motivated?

1. _____

2. _____

3. _____

4. _____

5. _____

Commit to taking action. You can't reach your new lifestyle if you think that *someday* you will be well. *Someday* you will start being clean. *Someday* is code for "never." Your someday has yet to come and will forever be this unnamed day. Turn *someday* into TODAY. Now.

There is power in setting up your intentions and installing them into your unconscious mind. Now that you know how this works, you will always be amazed at how much your life has shifted and changed for the better in light of this new knowledge.

KEY CONCEPTS:

ONGOING PROCESS

You need to continue to apply all that you have learned already in your daily life and continue to stay on top of your newly formed habits.

By committing to feeding your brain with positive information on a regular basis, you increase your daily level of motivation.

Choose the techniques you will use to stay motivated.

By writing down the specific and concrete actions you want to commit to, you are making yourself accountable.

You want to use all the tools you have learned so far to process these new commitments in your brain.

ABOUT THE AUTHORS

TOSCA RENO

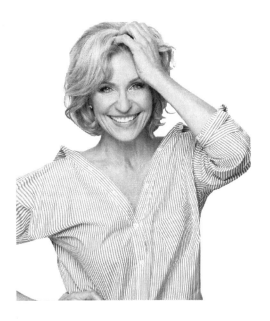

Photo credit: Liz Rosa, courtesy of Fresh Magazine

Tosca Reno is a New York Times bestselling author, founder of the Eat-Clean Diet® health revolution, health and wellness expert, transformation coach, motivational speaker, Star of a Gemini Award Winning reality TV show, physique competitor, and mother of 4.

Reno started her career at an age when most would consider retiring, earning her first Oxygen cover at 43, after losing 84 pounds and healing herself. She has competed in numerous physique contests and endurance events.

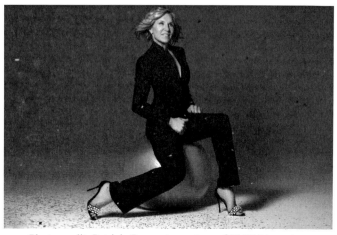

Photo credit: Patricia Recourt, courtesy of TMB Magazine.

The founder of the Eat Clean® series that kicked off a food revolution by the same name, Reno has sold millions of copies, in several languages. She has helped millions lose weight and become well, thanks to Eating Clean®. Once 204 pounds and officially obese, Reno has maintained this using the Eat Clean Diet® method.

Reno is best seen live, where she rivets the audience with her gut-wrenching authenticity. She loves life, and is a tenacious woman who has endured intense personal loss including the passing of her son, her husband and ultimately the family business and home. Reno is a force.

Reno is an expert health and wellness advisor for Canfitpro where she speaks, lectures and conducts wellness seminars and online education programs.

Often called "the woman with 9 lives," Reno has a depth of experience beyond many. Through her love of family she reveals her selflessness. Through her loss of love and child, she reveals her humanity. Through her consistent caring for others she shares her compassion. Through her grit she shows her resilience. When most would have given up, Reno still stands, sharing her smile and authenticity.

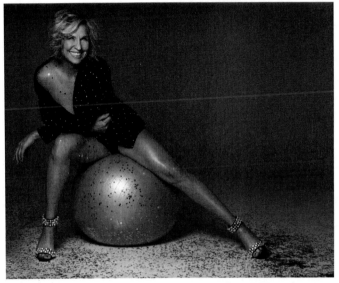

Photo credit: Patricia Recourt, courtesy of TMB Magazine.

Reno regularly contributes to various publications including Oxygen and Clean Eating.

She is currently developing a TV series with PBS, an episode of which will be aired in January/17.

Specialties: The psychology of overweight, motivation, inspiration, nutrition, exercise and one on one coaching.

Author, speaker, educator and media veteran.
www.toscareno.com
https://www.facebook.com/toscareno/
https://www.linkedin.com/in/tosca-reno-595831a6/

NATHALIE PLAMONDON-THOMAS

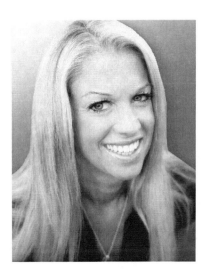

The Expert with a proven system to reprogram your brain and give you transformational results. Founder of the THINK Yourself® ACADEMY, speaker, Master Life Coach and No.1 best-selling author of seven books on wellness and empowerment. Nathalie combines over 25 years of experience in sales and over 30 years in the fitness industry. In 2007, Goodlife Fitness named her "Fitness Instructor of the Year" for Canada. She uses the principles of neuroscience and brain reprogramming in her practice as a Life Coach and Master Practitioner in NLP.

She retrains your brain to end self-sabotage and live your full potential. *"You can take a horse to water, but you can't make him drink"*. Somehow, Nathalie can.

"Hi, I'm Nathalie.

My parents were freaks!!!

They did not put a gate by the stairs when my brother and I were babies because they did not want to imply that we could fall. They didn't say: "Don't fall"; They would say: "Be careful around there." If they needed me to bring a full glass of water to the table, they would say: "Use a strong, firm hand and bring this glass to the table," instead of creating anxiety around the action of carrying the water by saying: "Don't spill it!"

There were signs everywhere in the house with motivational phrases like: "You can be everything you want"; "Yes you can"; "You will miss 100% of the shots you won't take"; "If you're going to do it, do it right", etc.

On Sundays, we didn't go to church (although we are Christian Catholics). Instead, my parents would make us sit in the living room to listen to motivational tape cassettes from Jean-Marc Chaput, Zig Ziglar, Og Mandino, etc. I was brainwashed into positive thinking at a very young age.

I believe that my life purpose is to motivate, inspire and support people to discover that they have everything inside themselves to be their best and live to their full potential.

I got my first 'calling' to help people at a very young age. My parents would not read us Disney stories at night. They would either sing us a song to put us to sleep with their guitar (which explains my love for music), or they would tell us motivational stories. Here is my favourite bedtime story: It is about an old man on the beach, who was throwing starfish back into the sea, one by one. A little girl asked him: "What are you doing sir?" and the old man responded: "I am saving the starfish from dying, as the tide brought them to shore, they will dry and die if I don't throw them back in the sea."

The little girl looked at the endlessly long beach and said: "But sir, no offence, but there are so many, you can't save them all! It doesn't really make a difference."

The old man responded, as he was showing the little girl the starfish that he was holding in his hands: "Well my dear, for this particular starfish, it makes a whole world of difference."

I was thinking: "When I grow up, I will be a starfish saviour and save them all, one at a time!" And the rest is history.

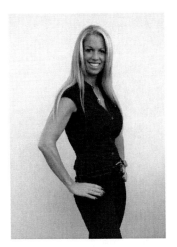

I was born in Saint-Raymond, a small town near Quebec City, Canada. I lived in Quebec for many years as a successful entrepreneur in the printing industry. I moved to Toronto, Ontario in my twenties, where I got seriously into fitness, personal training and nutrition consultation all while accumulating 16 more years of experience in sales in the natural food industry.

After reaching the top of my game as the No.1 Fitness Instructor in Canada, I realized that being my own personal best wasn't fulfilling me. I realized that even though I was helping people, my clients were not successful because I was giving them a better kale salad recipe or showing them a different way of doing push-ups. They thrived because they were changing the way they thought. Their mindset was influenced by mine.

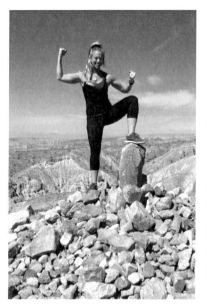

I then started to study neuroscience and the astonishing powers of the brain. I got a Neuro-Linguistic Programming (NLP) Master certification and Life Coaching certifications and have spent the last 10 years developing a system combining my experience as an entrepreneur, with my health and wellness knowledge and the specific processes I use with the thousands of clients I have helped to reach their full potential.

I work with clients one-on-one and propel people into the life they want through my coaching, books, events and speaking engagements. I also continue to teach fitness classes, 30 years and counting, using fitness as an introductory platform to help people be their best.

Eight years ago, I also started to work with children in schools, which gives me even more opportunity to impact and improve people's lives, as I believe if certain values are planted at a young age, flourishing happens sooner.

I now live in White Rock, British Columbia with my loving husband Duff and we are celebrating our 15th anniversary this year."

NATHALIE P.

Transformation Expert
Master Coach – No.1 Best Selling Author – Speaker – Publisher

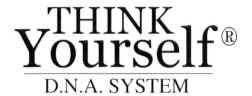

THINK Yourself®
D.N.A. SYSTEM

www.thinkyourself.com

https://www.facebook.com/nathalie.plamondonthomas

https://www.facebook.com/DNALifeCoaching/

https://www.linkedin.com/in/nathalie-plamondon-thomas-6b3262a/

twitter: @dnalifecoaching

From the same series:

THINK Yourself® SUCCESSFUL

THINK Yourself® THIN

THINK Yourself® HEALTHY

THINK Yourself® GRATEFUL

THINK Yourself® A RELATIONSHIP PRO

All available at: www.thinkyourself.com and www.amazon.com and www.amazon.ca

Coming out soon:

THINK Yourself® WEALTHY

THINK Yourself® AN AUTHOR

THINK Yourself® SEXY

THINK Yourself® SOBER

THANK YOU

Thank you to the following people who inspired me and contributed to this book:

Firstly, thank you TOSCA, co-author of THINK Yourself® CLEAN for the hours of meetings, planning, writing, strategizing, editing and laughing. We had a fun journey putting our respective experiences together. I have learned so much from you, and it has been an honour working with you. THINK Yourself® CLEAN is only the first of many projects we will accomplish together! Love you girl!

Thank you to my clients, for allowing me to be part of your journey, trusting me and causing me to grow as we walk together towards our life purpose. You keep me honest and on point. I am forever grateful to you.

Thank you to my parents Micheline and Yves Plamondon for your constant inspiration and support, and for being at the head of my 'fan-club'. You are always there for me and bring me so much energy.

Finally, thank you to my husband Duff Thomas for your continuous support and unconditional love. Once in a lifetime, you meet someone you want to share your soul with and despite them knowing everything about you, they love you anyways. Thank you, Duff. I love you too!

Nathalie